A Proven Plan to Ditch the Scale,
Get the Body You Want
& Wear the Clothes You Love!

DROP TWO SIZES

Rachel Cosgrove, BS, CSCS

RODALE.

© 2013 by Rachel Cosgrove

Photographs © Rodale Inc.

Rodale books may be purchased for business or promotional use or for special sales. For information, please write to: Special Markets Department, Rodale, Inc., 733 Third Avenue, New York, NY 10017

Women's Health is a registered trademark of Rodale Inc.

Printed in the United States of America
Rodale Inc. makes every effort to use acid-free ∞, recycled paper ♻.

Book design by Courtney Eltringham and Laura White
with George Karabotsos, design director of Men's Health and Women's Health Books

Photographs by Beth Bischoff
Real-Life Example photographs courtesy of participants

Library of Congress Cataloging-in-Publication Data is on file with the publisher.

ISBN 978-1-60961-463-8   paperback

Distributed to the trade by Macmillan
2   4   6   8   10   9   7   5   3   1   paperback

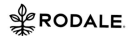

We inspire and enable people to improve their lives and the world around them.
rodalebooks.com

CONTENTS

ACKNOWLEDGMENTS

Thank you . . .

To the clients of Results Fitness—As a coach, nothing could be more fulfilling than being a part of your journey, coaching you through obstacles and doubts, watching you transform, then being there to experience the moment when you fit into your jeans and your face lights up in disbelief while exclaiming "They fit!" Thank you to every single client with whom I have had the opportunity to work closely. You are my inspiration. I love what I do!

To the Results Fitness team—Together we accomplished so much more than I ever could on my own. It is so incredible having a team who I consider my family to support me, to bounce ideas off of, to get feedback from, to use as guinea pigs, to learn from, to laugh and have fun with, and to be surrounded by every day—you are the most amazing, positive people. Every single one of you played a role in helping me create this book. A special thank you to Mike Wunsch and Craig Rasmussen, who are the masterminds behind the development of the programs at Results Fitness (including the one in this book) and Donna Bent, who reads everything I ever write (including this book) to make sure I look good. Thank you, team!

To our Mastermind Coaching Members of Results Fitness University—Many of you ran this exact system and shared the stories of your clients' successes, helping me to even further mold the plan laid out in this book. Together we are changing the way fitness is done!

To the fitness industry—There are so many professionals in this industry who have influenced me, guided me, taught me, and inspired me throughout my career. Thank you to all of them for continuing to elevate this industry. A special thank you to Chris Poirier for giving me the opportunity to share my passion on the Perform Better tour; Thomas Plummer for always pushing me to take the next step and encouraging me to put the proposal for this book together; and all of my colleagues, whom I consider friends, for your ongoing influence and support.

To Dr. Chris Mohr—Thank you for designing such easy-to-follow, delicious, effective menus for this book!

To Adam Campbell—Thank you for your encouragement and help with the proposal for this book and for the opportunity to shoot my first workout DVDs to go along with it! I really appreciate your support, helping me share what I'm passionate about.

To Ursula Cary, Jess Fromm, Marilyn Hauptly, Debbie McHugh, Angela Giannopoulos, George Karabotsos, Courtney Eltringham, Laura White, Allison Keane, and the rest of the team at Rodale Books—Thank you for bringing my book to life!

To Michele Promaulayko and Jen Ator—I'm so proud to have the *Women's Health* brand on this book. I love being a part of the WH team and appreciate the platform you give me to share my message with the WH audience.

To my mom—Thank you for being my best friend, my biggest supporter, and the most amazing mom there is.

To my dad—Thank you for introducing me to the gym all those years ago, being a strong role model throughout my life and always showing me how proud you are of me, which means more than you know.

To my grandma, my biggest fan—Thank you for being so much fun to share my accomplishments with. No one shows more excitement than you do!

To the rest of my family—Heather, Adam, Brent, Derek, Sandy, and, of course, Marie and John—You know me better than anyone and are all a part of my support team.

To Alwyn—Life is an adventure when you share it with the right person, and I'm having a blast on our adventure together!

To God—Throughout my life I have always leaned on my faith. I am absolutely blessed.

—Rachel Cosgrove

INTRODUCTION

Was it fairly easy to lose weight in the past, but now you can't shed a pound? Or worse, the more you try to lose weight, the more you seem to gain? Have you tried everything and still don't see results? Clients often come to me expressing their frustration that "nothing is working." They need a different approach to weight loss. And you might, too.

There may be a few reasons your previous plans haven't worked for you. After a lifetime of dieting, you have likely lost lean muscle each time you lost weight, slowing down your metabolism and making it harder and harder to see progress. This is especially true if you aren't seeing results after following low-calorie diets and weight loss plans that may have worked in the past.

Maybe you need different external feedback to monitor your progress. Up until now the scale has been the indicator of whether your diet or exercise program is working. If the scale doesn't budge, then you assume that your program must not be working. You think: I'm a failure. This is not true! And this cycle gets you nowhere closer to your goals.

By staying focused on the scale, you may be afraid of lifting weights and building muscle in fear that you will bulk up. But the fact is that your lean muscle mass, at this point, is most likely way below average. The only way to ever fit into your jeans again is to lift weights and gain lean body mass. This might keep that number on the scale from dropping as much as you are used to, but it will lead to an increased metabolism, which will reverse the damage you have done over a lifetime of dieting and—best of all—will lead to dropping two clothing sizes in just 8 to 12 weeks and completely reinventing your body. Now we're talking!

Excited? This is the feeling I want you to experience as you go through this book, which will tell you step by step exactly how to undo any damage from past diet plans and truly transform your body. Starting now, you will end the yo-yo diet trap and finally fit into your hottest wardrobe ever.

How This Plan Works

In August of 2009, our team launched a Skinny Jeans Challenge at our gym, Results Fitness, in Southern California. Working closely with our team of trainers, we watched as 20 women lost two jeans sizes in less than 12 weeks (most of them within 8 weeks). We've now run this challenge a number of times with consistent results. By following the very same program, you are guaranteed to drop two sizes in less than 12 weeks.

I have had women all over the United States follow the system and philosophies in this book, and they've all dropped two sizes. What's more, I have had coaches use this system at more than 50 gyms around the world—including gyms and clients in Switzerland, the Virgin Islands, Lebanon, Canada, and England—using this exact system and achieved the same results each time. This plan works! You'll read inspiring success stories from women all over the world who, just like you, wanted to transform their bodies—and they did.

The surprising thing, though, is that although my clients have dropped two sizes—for example, from a size 12 to a size 8—the average weight loss during these challenges has been only 4 pounds on the scale. I have even had a woman gain 2 pounds on the scale over the 12 weeks—and still drop two clothing sizes! My clients are always shocked and happy when they realize the scale no longer works as an indicator of how much fat they have lost.

Research at the Mayo Clinic published in *Obesity Journal* in May 2011 shows that weight loss does not equal fat loss. And two recent research studies from the United Kingdom and the Netherlands found clothing size to be an accurate indicator of your risk of health problems and disease. Clothes—not the scale—are the new indicator of health and fitness.

This book offers a proven, day-by-day solution to drop at least two sizes, fit into your favorite clothes in record time, and be able to maintain the results for the long term. Don't throw those skinny jeans out yet! Instead, throw out the scale and the fat clothes for good.

Are you ready to drop two sizes? Read on!

THIS TIME IS DIFFERENT

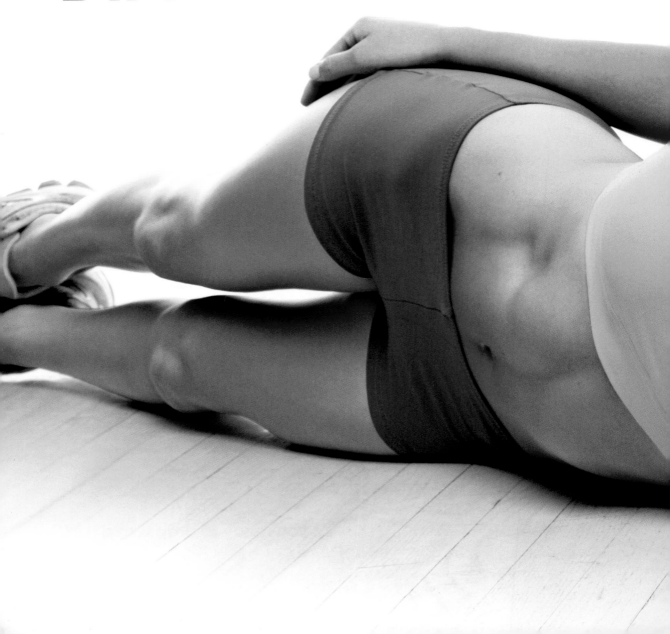

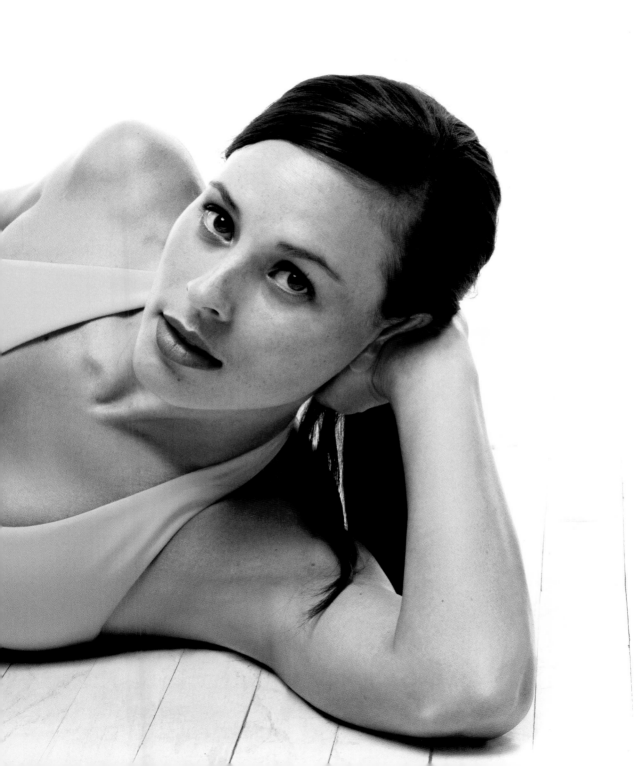

"The difference

is that I didn't just lose weight and get smaller; I actually changed my body. People don't ask me if I lost weight—they ask me if I have been working out. I feel empowered!"

—LISA ROUSSO, DROPPED FOUR SIZES

If you're like most women, you probably have three categories of clothing in your closet.

➜ *Your "skinny" clothes, which you refuse to throw out, even though you never wear them*

➜ *Your "fat" clothes, which you don't wear often, but keep around (even though their mere presence makes you so mad at yourself for rebounding from the last diet you were on)*

➜ *Your "in-between" clothes, which are probably the clothes you spend the most time wearing (except maybe when you're feeling bloated after the holidays and pull out your "fat" clothes for a while)*

Throughout your lifetime you have probably yo-yoed up and down, going on and off diets, struggling to be able to throw out all of your fat clothes for good. And the real dream? To one day have only "skinny" clothes in your closet. Sound familiar?

Does your "skinny" wardrobe include a pair of coveted "skinny" jeans that you now can't even get over your hips? Maybe one day you'll fit into them, but it seems so far away from where you are now. Are you wondering if you should give up and throw them out? Hang on!

A FALSE IDEAL

If you are, like the average woman, size 10 or above, you have probably been disappointed when shopping because most boutique and high-end fashion clothing stores don't cater to you. In fashion, size 14 is where plus-size starts, despite it being the size of the "average" woman. A *Los Angeles Times* article from 2009 titled "Fashion's Invisible Woman" said it perfectly:

> "When it comes to shopping, the average American man has it made. At 189.8 pounds and a size 44 regular jacket, he can wear Abercrombie & Fitch, American Apparel or Armani. Department stores, mall retailers and designer boutiques all cater to his physique—even when it's saddled with love handles, a sagging chest or a moderate paunch. In menswear, schlubby is accommodated. But the average US woman, who is 162.9 pounds and wears a size 14, is treated like an anomaly by apparel brands and retailers—who seem to assume that no one over size 10 follows fashion's capricious trends."

In a quest to fit into your skinny jeans and the fashionable apparel at most clothing stores, you may have considered going on a diet or doing whatever will work to look and feel the way you want to. But this "ideal" often leads to disaster. Three out of every four American women between the ages of 25 and 45 report having disordered eating behaviors, according to a survey from the University of North Carolina at Chapel Hill. Dieting this way leads to temporary weight loss and a focus on hitting the magic number on the scale. You may have hit this magic number in the past and bought yourself a pair of fashionable jeans in your new size—your "skinny" jeans. The problem is that the majority of the weight loss you achieved was likely from reduced lean muscle mass, the loss of which slows down your metabolism—and keeping your metabolism humming is one of the keys to lasting weight loss.

You may have been on this roller-coaster ride, even recently, and already gained pounds back at this point, returning to the weight you were originally or even getting heavier. Your size 12 or 14 jeans (now known as your "fat" jeans) may fit even worse because your body is now made up of more fat and less muscle.

First, know this: You're not alone. This yo-yo phenomenon is very common among women, and many times the process is repeated over and over for a lifetime. A study conducted in Australia in 2009 suggested that women ages 25 to 45 (most of you reading this book) are at the highest risk of gaining weight, and those with children are at increased risk because of weight gain associated with pregnancy and subsequent lifestyle changes. The study noted that average self-reported weight gain is almost 1½ pounds per year. From 25 to 45, that adds up! The goal of this challenge is to reverse that.

You may have a number on the scale associated with those skinny clothes, which you have reached before—it's where you think you have to be in order to look and feel the way you want to. Throughout your lifetime, you may have reached this magic number on the scale more than once by following various crash diets and plans, but each time the results were fleeting, as the pounds slowly crept back on.

A restrictive diet sets you up to fail. A study published in the *New England Journal of Medicine* in 2011 looked at the long-term hormonal effects of weight loss from a low-calorie diet. The results showed the damage was still evident a year later, with a number of hormones still affected, including appetite control hormones. You'll still feel hungrier and more likely to binge a whole year after you've finished your low-calorie diet. It is impossible to maintain your weight loss when your body is fighting you to gain the weight back even a whole year later. A different approach—this one—that includes exercise, fueling your body with the right foods, and not focusing on weight loss will set you up to succeed.

Every time you've reached your magic number on the scale, you have most likely lost muscle, which slows down your metabolism and makes it harder and harder to ever fit into those "skinny" clothes. Each time you crash dieted, you exchanged muscle for fat, changing the way you look for the worse and slowing your metabolism more and more.

THE EMOTIONAL COST OF DIETING

Going through these ups and downs not only changes your shape, but it's also an emotional roller coaster. Each time you gain back the weight, you feel like a failure, and so begins the negative dialogue. I'm a failure. I have no willpower. I'll never be thin. Beating yourself up does nothing but make your self-esteem plummet, kill your confidence, and cast a hopeless pall on the idea of getting in shape.

When the scale tops out at your limit (or maybe it's when you can no longer zip up that trusty black dress), you jump on a crash diet that seemed to work before.

You'll weigh yourself each week, or worse, each day, letting the scale decide whether you will be in a good mood or a bad mood that day. At this point, however, the scale doesn't budge like it used to, making the entire process more frustrating.

You may have added exercise into the equation, usually in the form of aerobics, including walking or running, in which calories are burned but lean body mass is not built. Once again, the body will break down muscle as a form of fuel.

After this cycle of dieting, weight loss, skinny jeans, weight gain, and the return to fat jeans, the average woman is still a size 14 or higher, doesn't fit into her "skinny" clothes, and has slowed her metabolism down because her lean muscle mass is now practically nonexistent. Now, the same diets that worked before to get into those smaller clothes no longer work. Does this sound like you?

As the years go by, it gets harder and harder to reach this magic number, especially with increasing demands on your schedule, family, career, and other stresses. Your body no longer responds like it used to. Even the strictest diet doesn't work like it did in the past. This is discouraging, and you may feel like you will never look and feel the way you want to and above all, never fit into your favorite clothes again.

Why Muscle Matters

Does adding or losing muscle really affect your metabolism?

YES! There have been research studies that have shown an increase of anywhere from 6 calories a day up to 50 calories a day burned for 1 pound of muscle added. With the type of strength training programs you'll be doing, you'll notice a boost of closer to 50 calories a day burned per pound of muscle gained, although it makes more sense to look at the body and metabolism as a whole rather than how many calories 1 pound of muscle burns (since it is impossible to use that 1 pound on its own). Researcher Wayne Westcott, PhD, CSCS, instructor in the exercise science department at Quincy College in Massachusetts, wrote an excellent article comparing the different studies that have been done and concluded that the 6-calories-a-day equation is inaccurate and that it could be closer to 35 calories. He showed that with a very basic strength program (not the cutting-edge protocol you'll find in this book), the average person gains about 3 pounds of muscle over 3 months and increases his or her resting metabolism by about 7 percent. With this program I have seen women gain much more than 3 pounds of muscle in 3 months. Their average weight loss is 4 pounds, but they lose 2 clothing sizes—or more!

THROW OUT THE SCALE!

Working with hundreds of women over the years, I have realized that women need external feedback when we're working to transform our bodies. When we look into a mirror, it is very hard for us to see positive changes because we're usually so focused on our own flaws.

Research shows that women are much more critical of themselves than men are when it comes to evaluating their own appearance. In fact, statistics have shown that 8 out of 10 women are dissatisfied with their reflections in the mirror, many seeing distorted images of themselves no matter how much they're changing. (Most women look back at pictures of themselves and simply think, "I was fat," not, "What a great family vacation. I looked really fit in those hiking shorts!") Over their lifetimes, since they can't count on the mirror, women have learned that the scale will tell them if their bodies are changing or not. Women give the scale too much power because it is the only definitive indicator they seem to have. "If the scale says X, I am where I want to be," they reason.

Taking the focus off of the scale and off of the mirror and onto how your clothes fit improves body image because

you see the changes happening right before your eyes. A 2011 study conducted at the Technical University of Lisbon in Lisbon, Portugal, was done with 239 women over 12 months working on improving their body image. As the participants improved their body image, eating self-regulation became easier. We have to take a different approach than stepping on the scale, which only results in destructive, negative mind-sets leading to poor body image and making it harder to change habits long term.

If you're ready to take a completely different approach—one that has been proven to work over and over again to help hundreds of women—and drop two sizes in 12 weeks, this book is for you! But there's one catch: You are not allowed to step on a scale. The scale is no longer a valid indicator of whether your body is changing. In fact, it's one of the primary culprits behind you not reaching your potential physically and mentally.

This book is laid out as a challenge, not a diet. As you'll see below, there's a big difference!

A Diet

→ You go "on" a diet, like a switch, eventually turning "off" the diet.

→ A diet is not something you plan to do long term. It is strict, extreme, and meant to get results, not let you have a life.

→ You aim for a number on the scale. Once you hit that number, the diet is over.

→ It doesn't matter what you lose, as long as the scale goes down and you hit the "magic number."

→ If you do have a weak moment and go "off" your diet, it usually leads to beating yourself up and a spiral of destructive behaviors as you continue to "blow your diet."

A Challenge

→ You will change old habits and build new behaviors each day and week until they are part of your daily regimen.

→ The challenge may feel tough at first, but after the first 30 days, your new behaviors will become a way of life.

→ Your daily routine can be flexible. The first research study to evaluate self-regulation with weight loss and weight maintenance over 2 years, conducted at the Technical University of Lisbon, showed that one of the keys to sustained results is to end emotional eating (the "on" and "off" pattern) and instead allow flexibility to realistically stick to your new lifestyle long-term. You'll learn about the 90 percent rule and how to enjoy splurging when you choose to.

→ The challenge is a kick start to thinking differently about yourself, your weight, your health, and the rest of your life—as the new you.

Think of this challenge as a journey, like driving from Point A to Point B. At first it may feel familiar, like starting the ignition of your car. The difference is that this time you'll finally reach your destination. Point B is that glorious moment when you slide on those hot, super-flattering jeans and step out looking and feeling fabulous—for the rest of your life. The key is that the end of this book is not the end of your journey!

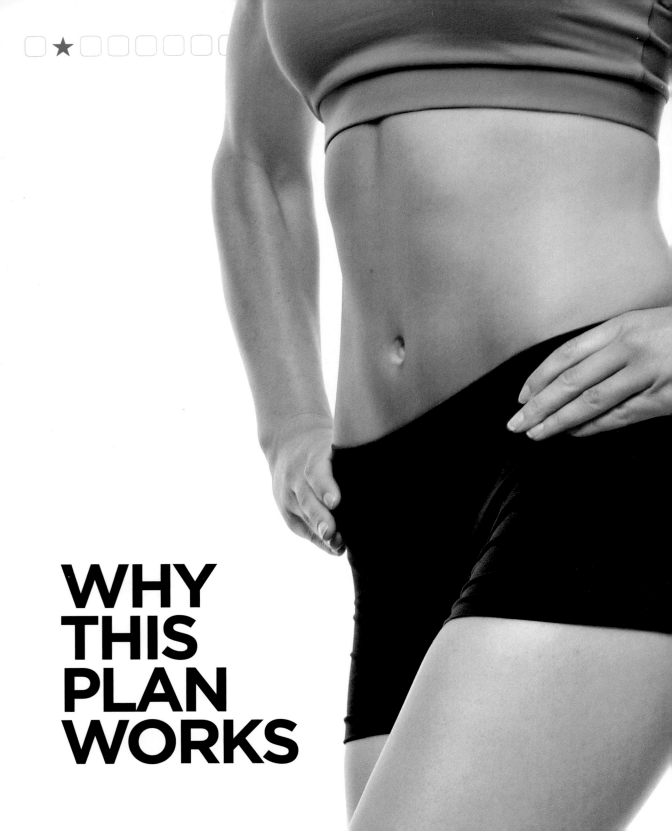

WHY THIS PLAN WORKS

"I can give you solid reasons (excuses) as to why I shouldn't have committed to Drop Two Sizes: I work full time; I'm getting ready to go back to school; I have four kids and a new puppy; and I recently quit smoking. But now that my jeans fit I know I can do anything I put my mind to. I can't wait to take on life's journey at full speed."

—LISA OLWELL, DROPPED TWO SIZES IN 8 WEEKS

When my first book came out, I had already started to use clothes as a measurement for weight loss. I used the phrase "Your Thermometer Jeans," which told you when you're hot and when you're not. I ran the first official Jeans Challenge right after I wrote my first book and watched as every single one of the participants dropped two clothing sizes! I also realized how useless the scale is as a way to measure your weight loss progress. So many faces lit up as women went through the challenge and saw their bodies shrink before their eyes when they fueled their bodies with the right foods and lifted weights. I knew I had something I wanted to share on a broader level. Since then I have taken hundreds of women through the challenge and have landed on some very significant findings.

YOU WILL SHRINK, EVEN IF THE SCALE DOESN'T BUDGE

Really? The scale doesn't move and you shrink? Absolutely. I have tracked the progress of hundreds of women (some of whose stories are featured in this book) and have seen over and over again instances where the scale doesn't budge— but they dropped two sizes and fit into a whole new wardrobe.

How can that be? If you have lost muscle from a weight loss program or crash diet in the past, you probably have below-average lean body mass. Your body needs to build muscle to be healthier and, yes, thinner. Because of this, your body will respond to strength training by dramatically increasing your lean muscle in a very short period of time while at the same time losing fat.

A study done at Queen's University in Canada tracked 54 women in four groups: Group one dieted and lost weight; group two exercised and lost weight; group three exercised without weight loss; and group four was a weight-stable control. The women who exercised and did not lose weight lost the same amount of fat as the diet group who did lose weight. The difference? The exercise group now had added lean muscle that makes keeping the fat off much easier in the long term, along with being fitter at the end of the study. The study concluded that exercise without weight loss is associated with a *substantial reduction* in total and abdominal obesity. The numbers on the scale do not have to go down to lose fat and get smaller!

YOU'LL GET SLIM AND TONED, NOT BULKY

I used to tell female clients who were afraid of bulking up not to worry about gaining muscle. I'd explain that their bodies wouldn't gain muscle as easily as a man's because they didn't have the same levels of testosterone. But I was wrong: They *needed* to gain muscle in order to transform their bodies. I would take a client's body fat percentage. It would often be fairly high, with relatively low muscle (which is probably why they hired a trainer!). As they started the program, their body fat percentage would start to come down, even though the scale wouldn't budge. This often caused frustration, and I heard many times that women didn't want to gain muscle. Guess what? Women do gain muscle and, in order to tone up and slim down, they *should!* In fact, most women have such a low percentage of muscle to begin with that gaining just 10 pounds of muscle will get them up to normal levels, fire up their metabolisms, and help them shed fat to reveal the bodies they want and keep them long-term.

In a research study in Denmark, 27 participants on a calorie-restricted diet without exercise lost, on average, 19 pounds in 8 weeks, or about 2.38 pounds a week (this is typical of most weight loss programs). Only 68 percent of it was from fat. The other 32 percent was lean muscle mass. For every 13 pounds of fat lost, they also gave up 6 pounds of metabolically active muscle. Extrapolating this out over 12 weeks would mean a loss of 24 pounds total: 16 pounds from fat and almost 8 from muscle. Most women have done more than one calorie-restricted diet in their lifetimes, so multiplying that by two means they have lost 16 pounds of muscle (and that's only from two diet plans). How many calorie-restricted diets have you embarked on in your lifetime?

What does this mean? Your goal is to get your lean body mass, or muscle—the very thing you are terrified of building because you don't want to get too "big and bulky"—to start increasing as fast as possible in order to get your normal metabolism back, which will help transform your body. This is exactly what will happen during this challenge, which is why you are not allowed to watch the scale.

Clothing size—not the scale—has also been proven as an accurate indicator of your overall health. Research studies in the United Kingdom looked at a number of health markers without looking at the scale and found that women who wear larger clothing sizes (over a size 16) are at an increased risk for health problems such as

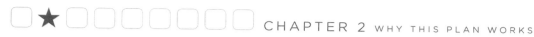
heart disease, cardiovascular disease, cancer, and diabetes. Clothing size is the new health and fitness indicator, not the scale.

YOU'LL BE MOTIVATED TO ACHIEVE REAL RESULTS

If I'm taking your scale away, how will you know if you're making progress? You are probably used to starting a diet and watching the pounds melt off on the scale. This is what you've been programmed to use as your indicator of progress. As I've mentioned previously, it's also exactly what got you in this situation in the first place—some of those pounds melting off are actually metabolically active muscle. But when nothing else is working, it's time to do something completely different.

In general, women need external feed-back when it comes to changing our bodies. Now that you know the scale is no longer a useful tool, how else will you see your body's improvement? You could look in the mirror, but this isn't an accurate tool either. Most of us look in the mirror and see every flaw, no matter how much weight we've actually lost or how toned we've become. I see it over and over again. How many of you have "felt" fat at some point in your life, then looked back

at pictures and realized you really looked fantastic? At the time you couldn't celebrate your accomplishment because you were focused on the negative. Research has shown that women who focus on themselves in the mirror can develop a negative body image, and other research confirmed that what women see in the mirror is unrelated to their percentage of body fat (meaning that women with less body fat may see a reflection that they view as having higher amounts).

The mirror will not work to measure your progress, and neither will the scale. This is why this book is different—and how it will help you finally succeed in creating the body you crave. Your clothes are the best, most accurate measurement of how much your body is changing. Clothes don't lie. They either fit or they don't! And you will get smaller and fitter, despite what the scale says or what you see in the mirror.

YOU'LL NEVER YO-YO DIET AGAIN

A woman and her 19-year-old daughter joined our program. After a few weeks, the daughter had lost pounds on the scale but the mother had not. Frustrated, the mother wanted to know why her daughter was losing weight but she wasn't. I asked her how many diets or weight loss programs she'd done in her lifetime, and she replied, "Hundreds. You name it, I've done it." How about the daughter? She had never dieted before; in fact, this was her first time joining an exercise program. She had never gone on a calorie-restricted diet and lost precious muscle mass, only to gain the weight back—while her mom had repeated this cycle, in her words, "hundreds of times" (or at least, quite a few).

If you think back to what we discussed earlier in this chapter, you'll realize that losing muscle mass "hundreds of times" adds up to a *lot* of lean muscle lost and a sluggish metabolism. But as soon as she joined my program, the mom started fueling her body properly and lifting weights, restoring her metabolism and getting fit. It just wasn't showing up on the scale.

There is an inverse relationship between the number of diets and weight loss programs a woman has done in her lifetime, and the amount the scale will go down when she starts one of my programs. The more crash diets or weight loss programs you've done over your lifetime, the less likely the scale will budge. But that's okay!

Research conducted by the Mayo Clinic in May 2011 showed that weight loss does *not* equal improved body composition— in other words, just because the scale goes down doesn't mean you have less body fat. Their results showed that improvement in body composition may go undetected in almost one-third of people whose weight remained the same and in one-third of people who gained weight. That's a lot of people who walked out feeling like they failed because the scale went up or stayed the same, even though their body composition had actually improved. The scale is no longer a valid indicator. Get rid of it!

In addition, a research study conducted at the University of Nebraska showed that by adding strength training, even with a calorie deficit, you can gain muscle. This study put participants on an 800-calorie-per-day liquid diet (note: I do not recommend this) along with a strength training program, for 90 days. The average weight loss over the 90-day period was 35 pounds, and all of the participants increased their amount of muscle significantly because they included strength training. Adding muscle helped them look more defined as they lost weight, rather than getting smaller—but still flabby. This shows that weight training can increase muscle mass (and therefore boosts metabolism) even during severe energy restriction and large-scale weight loss. Remember: Even if the scale doesn't budge, you can get smaller and gain muscle at the same time.

YOU'LL THINK AHEAD, PLAN AHEAD

Pull out your calendar and look over the next 12 weeks. What do you have coming up? Any vacations? Special events? Anything preplanned that you'll need to strategize around to be able to commit 100 percent? Mark on your calendar anything you will need to pay special attention to so that you can fully dive into this plan, no matter what the circumstances. Highlight any events you are looking forward to where you can start rocking your new clothes! Visualizing yourself in a hot outfit or with energy to burn will keep you motivated and provide an important benchmark for success.

The day-by-day road maps beginning on page 52 are laid out for the entire 12-week challenge. Flip to that section and check it out to get an idea of what you are committing to. Days 1 through 84 are explained in detail so you can mentally prepare. I recommend photocopying the Workout Calendar starting on page 29 and posting it above your desk or in your kitchen. You'll start to enjoy seeing all those days crossed off as you get closer to wearing your favorite jeans or dress!

Each day you will focus on a habit. While I ask you to focus on only one per day, over time, you'll start to build patterns of positive action. These seemingly small tasks will snowball into a lifetime of healthy behavior—not to mention the ability to wear anything you like! I will include a checklist each day, including actions like:

→ *Get psyched by visualizing yourself in your skinny jeans.*

→ *Challenge yourself with the workout for that day, whether it is a strength workout, a metabolic workout, an interval workout, or a day off.*

→ *Plan ahead for your meals: Figure out your next 24 hours and pencil in what you plan to eat in your journal.*

YOU'LL COMMIT TO MOVE

While it's possible to lose weight without exercising, this plan specifically uses strength training to build lean muscle and transform your body. You will need to move—but I promise, you'll enjoy it! Now that you have thought through your next 12 weeks, decide realistically how many days a week you can commit to working out. Keep in mind that this plan is designed to be somewhat flexible to fit in with your lifestyle. You must commit to a minimum of 3 days a week to get results, but I strongly recommend you commit to 4 days a week if you can.

Compared to sedentary women, active women tend to have lower body fat and significantly higher resting metabolic rates. Commit to moving as often as you can while also allowing for recovery. You will have active recovery days, where you will continue to be active in a way that will still allow your body to recover.

Take a minute to write down this sentence in your journal or post it where you can see it every day:

"I commit to working out ____ days a week and will do whatever it takes to make that happen."

YOU'LL BANISH THE WORD *BUT*

One of the biggest challenges many women face is actually the simplest exercise of all: end all negative body-bashing thoughts and excuses. Any time you use the word *but* you have completely discounted whatever commitment you just made to yourself. For example: "I am going to cook at home this week, *but* I don't know if that will work because we have a really busy week." You put a good intention forth and then took it right back with that pesky word but. BUT stands for Behold the Underlying Truth. Instead, practice using the word *and*.

Tips to Keep Committed

REMEMBER THAT FIT CHICKS OF A FEATHER FLOCK TOGETHER.

Find a friend to support you or even join you. Make dates to work out together and keep each other accountable. Swap your favorite goal clothes for extra motivation. Social support is very important. A 1999 study done in Pennsylvania looked at the benefits of increased social support for weight loss and maintenance and determined that those who recruited friends had better results at the end of the 4-month study, along with an increased chance of maintaining their weight loss for the long-term.

THROW OUT YOUR FAT CLOTHES.

Put a box in your closet or bedroom to start to throw clothes into as they get too big for you. Over the course of the plan, when you pull something out of your closet and realize it is too baggy, toss it into the box. At the end of the 12 weeks you can take the box to Goodwill or another charity.

GET A JOURNAL TO KEEP TRACK OF YOUR PROGRESS.

Get a journal specifically for this plan and keep track of your daily nutrition, your thoughts, and your workouts. Tracking your progress will keep you motivated and accountable.

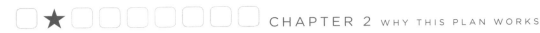

"I am going to cook at home this week, *and* we have a really busy week." Now those two things can coexist. Instead of discounting the good intention, your brain recognizes that you need to come up with a solution to the issue of cooking during a busy week.

Other offenders? Try, kinda, and sorta. Start to catch yourself anytime you use one of these words. All you're doing is giving yourself an excuse and undermining your progress. "I'll try to get to the gym three times this week." How about you *will*? Start to change your patterns and soon it'll become easier to stay on track.

When I ask, "Are you following the nutrition rules and menus from the plan"? I often hear, "Most of the time." What I have consistently seen is that when a client says "most of the time," she is following my advice about 70 percent of the time. Now, 70 percent may feel like "most of the time," but the truth is that it's not enough to see results. This means it is time to bump up your efforts to achieve 90 percent— or "almost all of the time." It's that extra effort that will make all the difference.

YOU'LL TAKE THE VOW

A 12-week study conducted at Florida State University in 2011 with 109 overweight participants looked at the consequences of focusing on the goals they were working to achieve for the entire 12 weeks, compared to a group who focused on the progress they had already made while pursuing a weight loss goal. The group who focused on their goals was twice as successful. They reported higher levels of commitment to their goals and ultimately lost more weight.

Pull out the pair of jeans or the cute little black dress you are going to work toward fitting into and hang it somewhere within easy reach. Imagine yourself getting into it without a struggle. Now, take a "before" picture of yourself. As you'll see in so many of the inspiring stories in this book, a photo truly can say a thousand words—and you'll be happily surprised when you reach your goal and have the evidence to prove it! After you take the picture, sit down with the following words and say them out loud:

"I vow that over the next 12 weeks, I will not step foot on a scale or body fat machine. I will not count calories. I will only use my clothing as my measurement. I will fuel my body with the right foods and challenge myself with the workouts. I promise that I will only say nice things to myself throughout the 12 weeks. I will trust this plan."

During this plan, if you ever feel lost or discouraged, come back to this vow and repeat it out loud. Remind yourself why you want to drop two sizes, and how hard you've already worked to get there. Come back to your mission statement (see below) for an extra push toward success. You *can* achieve the results you want!

YOU'LL FIND A MISSION STATEMENT

What will drive you to stay focused and on track? When you have a weak moment (and they do happen, as we all know), having a mission statement or mantra can give you a much-needed boost. Part of dropping two sizes and fitting back into your clothes is getting comfortable with the uncomfortable feeling you'll surely have as you start to change your habits. This saying will get you through those moments.

You'll read some of these in the powerful testimonials in this book: "Now is my time"; "Only I can decide to get closer to my goal"; "Nothing tastes as good as two sizes smaller feels"; "Be strong, be fit, be confident"; "The best of me is yet to come"; and "Steady goodness."

Nike coined the most famous slogan, "Just Do It!" They make fitness apparel with other inspiring phrases that make my workouts a little more fun and energized. I have T-shirts that say, "Doing It!" and "Strong Is the New Beautiful!" and "I Got Your Woman Power Right Here!"

Come up with your own and write it here, and also in your journal. Refer to it as many times as you need to throughout this journey!

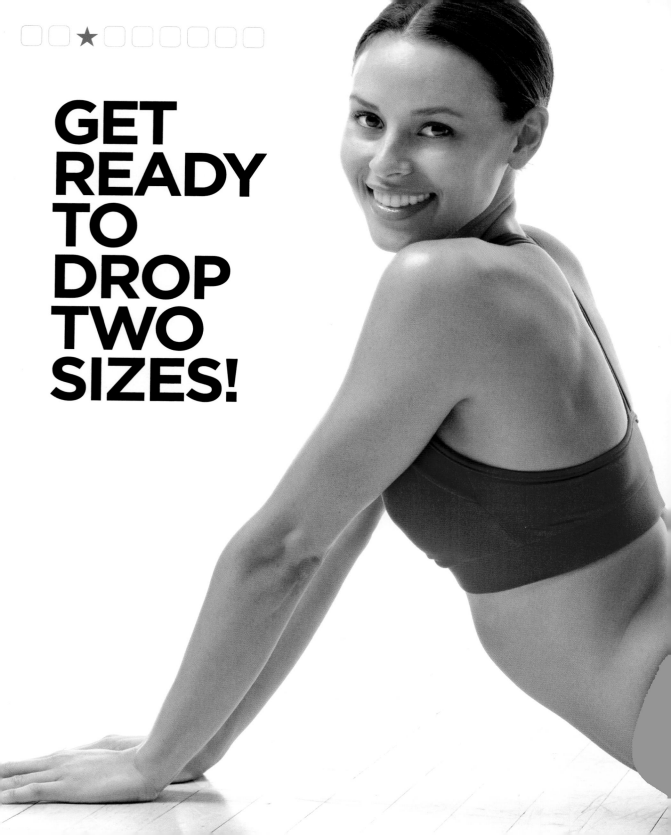

GET
READY
TO
DROP
TWO
SIZES!

"I finally got real.

I got honest with myself and realized that if I was going to achieve my goal and get my body back, it would mean saying NO more often and YES to myself. I made my gym time sacred and scheduled. I made a commitment to myself, and I wouldn't allow anything to derail my workout time."

—CINDY SCHEER, DROPPED TWO SIZES IN 8 WEEKS

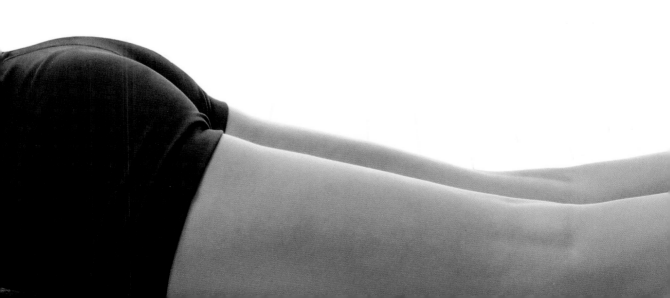

This book is designed as a road map that will guide you through exactly what to do in order to drop two sizes over the next 12 weeks. There are three phases, and in each phase, you'll find a step-by-step weekly plan, along with the workouts and the menus you'll need.

In the following chapters, you'll learn how to start your journey, including setting up your workout routine, making sure you have the proper equipment, cleaning out your kitchen and stocking up on healthy options, and starting to track your progress in a journal.

The recommendations on this road map are not randomly chosen. I took careful notes while guiding real people through this exact challenge—so I know what questions you might ask, and when you will need some extra motivation. I have now run dozens of these challenges, each with 20 to 50 people who have all had success following this exact system—just look at some of their amazing success stories to know you're in good company! In addition, I have had a number of fitness coaches also use this system successfully with their clients. Bottom line: It works! All you need to do is follow the map, and you'll drop two sizes (at least)—guaranteed.

HOW TO FOLLOW THE WEEKLY PLAN—CHECK!

Throughout this journey you will see the following checkpoints, which are daily behaviors you will adopt to successfully reach your goal. You may be used to writing down your weight each day or week from a past weight loss program. This time, you'll write down what you wore that made you feel fabulous, sexy, or great about yourself— much more fun, in my opinion! It might be a new hat or pair of shoes in the beginning, but soon enough you'll be rocking your slimmest jeans and the rest of your favorite clothes. Every day, choose to wear something that makes you feel good and jot it down in your journal.

These checkpoints will serve as reminders:

Attitude Check ✓

Attitude is everything, especially as you go through the next 12 weeks. Part of the challenge is to teach your mind to work positively. Focus on expecting success and eliminate any negative thinking. This is key to your progress these next 12 weeks. Evidence shows that incorporating mind-set checks along with nutrition and exercise enhances results. Throughout the challenge you will have Attitude Checkpoints to check in with yourself and make sure you are heading in the right direction when it comes to shifting your mind-set.

Splurge Check

You can get away with enjoying a splurge 10 percent of the time. If you are eating four to five meals a day, this is equal to three meals a week. For this challenge, make it a goal to plan out your splurges and indulge a maximum of three times a week. If you are following the plan 90 percent of the time, you'll see results. You must track your food in a journal in order to stay on target. Please don't rely on your memory!

Throughout the challenge, you'll have a Splurge Check when you'll take inventory of how many splurges on average you have had over the entire challenge up to that point. If you are averaging three a week (maybe you had four one week and two the next), you are in good shape. If you are averaging more than three, it is time to make up that average. If you get too far off the path, all is not lost! Just regroup and get back to the road map as soon as possible.

Jeans Check

Every 3 weeks throughout the challenge, you'll have a Jeans Check. As we've discussed, your clothes are truly the best measurement of your transformation. I use jeans as the primary example, but any pair of pants or fitted skirt can also serve as your checkpoint clothing item. The goal is to drop two sizes, so choose something that realistically fits this plan—even if you end up dropping more. No matter how much you may not want to, try on this item of clothing every 3 weeks to keep track of your progress. This is what you might expect:

Week One: They don't fit at all, maybe not even over your thighs. (Don't despair: They will fit soon, I promise!)

Week Three: They can get over your hips already! And even if you can't zip or button them, you're close.

Week Six: With some force, you can get them zipped! It may not be pretty (or comfortable), but they're on! This is the halfway point.

Week Nine: You can probably wear your jeans by now. Depending on your progress, they may still be a bit tight or be very close to comfortable.

Week Twelve: Slide them on and strut your stuff! You may even need a new pair to show off your figure!

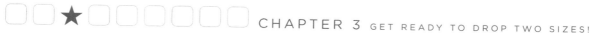

Water Check

Throughout the 12 weeks, make it a priority to drink water. Think of water as your fat-burning liquid. Replace all beverages with water if you can, and make it a goal to get a minimum of 64 ounces—or 8 glasses—each day. If you are not hydrated, your body will not perform optimally and you will not get the same results. Water also helps keep your skin glowing.

Keep in mind that all fluids count, outside of alcohol, so if plain water isn't your thing, you can count green tea, seltzer, or any other beverage toward that 8-glass total. Keep in mind these drinks should be calorie free and, ideally, not artificially sweetened. If you get bored with plain water, add sliced fruit or veggies (cucumber is refreshing) to keep it fun and flavorful.

De-Stress Check

Throughout the 12 weeks, another habit you'll work on is how to take at least 10 minutes each day to de-stress. This is crucial in order to lower the levels of your stress hormone, cortisol, and let your body decompress. High cortisol levels have been linked to high belly fat. You'll be asking a lot of your body on this plan, and it's important to give yourself a chance to rest and reboot. This check will remind you to take at least 10 minutes every day to do one of the following (or come up with your own relaxing ritual):

→ *Close your eyes in silence and practice deep breathing.*

→ *Take a hot bath or sit in the steam room at your gym.*

→ *Stretch or do yoga poses on your own, in silence.*

→ *Get a pedicure, massage, or facial— you deserve it!*

→ *Take a leisurely walk outside, or sit peacefully in a place that relaxes you.*

Veggie Check

One of the biggest challenges for most people is to eat enough vegetables— and a *variety* of vegetables. You should eat a fruit or a vegetable at each meal, with a goal in Phase One of including at least three servings of vegetables every day, working up to 10. Check out the nutrition section starting on page 80 for easy, delicious recipe ideas for meals and snacks. Remember that a serving size is only about the size of your fist, so a large salad can easily count as three or even four servings. Veggies fill you up and provide valuable nutrients, helping you stay satisfied while slimming down.

Posture Check

Don't slouch. Sit up straight!

Okay, how many of you just reacted by throwing your shoulders back and sitting or standing at attention? Slouching or slumping over is something we're all guilty of doing, whether we're hunched over our computers at work, the steering wheel of a car, or the treadmill at the gym. Good posture doesn't just make you look taller and more confident; it helps strengthen your postural muscles, which support a straight, slim figure. Throughout the challenge, you'll have a Posture Check. As you build up strength, good posture will come more naturally.

Brake Check

As you continue through the plan, you'll start to improve other aspects of your life—maybe you'll gain more energy, have deeper sleep, experience reduced joint pain, or even enjoy a more fulfilling sex life! But as you step on the accelerator toward these goals, you may feel your progress suddenly halted by one of three main areas I call the brakes: nutrition, exercise, or your attitude. It's extremely personal, and only you will know which one you'll struggle with the most.

Be aware of which one (or combination) puts the brakes on your progress.

For example, are you constantly missing workouts? Are you slipping on your nutrition? Or do you continually put yourself down no matter how well you've followed the plan? Record these speed bumps in your journal and make a conscious effort to push past them.

Sleep Check

Getting enough sleep seems to be the biggest challenge for many people. The common recommendation of 8 hours per night holds true, although some people will need slightly more or less. Without enough sleep, your energy levels will plummet, so you'll tend to crave sugar (which further affects your energy levels and mood), and you won't be able to optimally perform during your workouts or recover from them properly.

When you sleep, your body regenerates and rebuilds. You are asking a lot of your body over the next 12 weeks, so reward yourself by making a restful night's sleep a priority! Your Sleep Checks are there to remind you to set yourself up for beneficial z's.

THE WORKOUTS

"**It is really** easy to become lazy and to forget what it really feels like to be strong and healthy. If there is something that you want to change about yourself, don't wait another minute. You might need to make major life changes to get healthy, figure out how to do it, and find someone to support and encourage you. I have learned that women can be really strong and look amazing!"

—STACY LUNDBERG, DROPPED FROM A SIZE 24 TO A SIZE 12

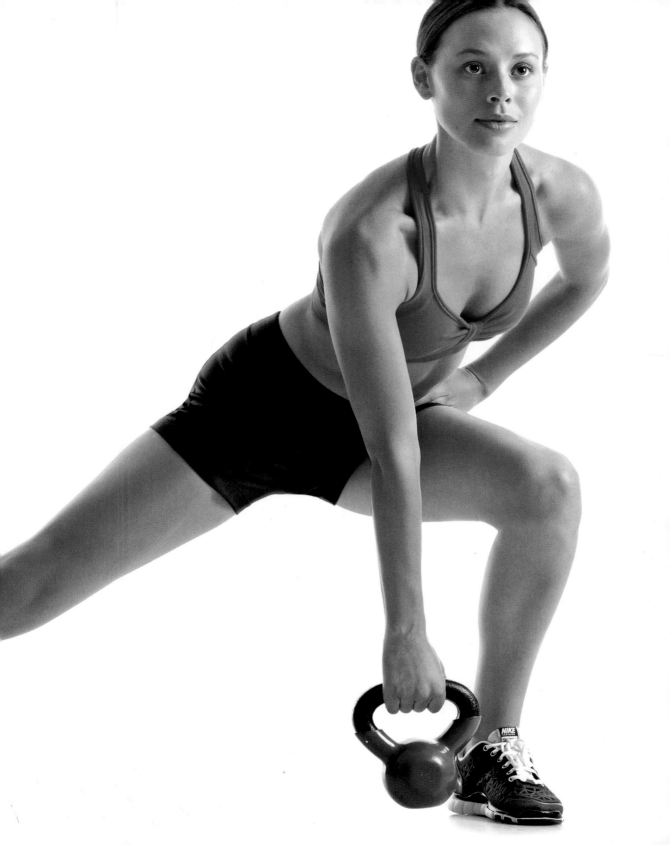

The exercise plan laid out in this book is based on the exact programs we use at Results Fitness. I worked closely with Mike Wunsch, CSCS, and Craig Rasmussen, CSCS, to design and deliver the most effective plan possible—which you now hold in your hands! Between the three of us, we have written thousands of programs, trained hundreds of women every year, and tracked every result. This plan is based on what works.

Before you jump into the workouts, make sure you have everything you need to succeed.

SHOULD YOU JOIN A GYM?

If there is a gym in your area that is convenient, affordable, and has the equipment and/or classes you need, by all means, join! It's worth the investment to have a place to go to escape the distractions at home to do your workout, especially if the environment is friendly and supportive.

What should you look for? You don't need rooms full of equipment to sit on. Make sure the gym has the following:

→ *Dumbbells and/or kettlebells*

→ *A cable system with adjustable height settings*

→ *A TRX suspension trainer*

→ *A bench and/or a step*

→ *A mat*

→ *A foam roller, lacrosse ball, or The Stick to massage your muscles. These tools work great to give your muscles a quick massage without having to fork out the big bucks for a masseuse.*

You'll usually find most of this in a corner where the trainers spend most of their time with their clients. It's a bonus if you have access to barbells, plates, and a power rack, which most gyms should have.

In addition, you may want to purchase one or two kettlebells or pairs of dumbbells so you can do your metabolic workouts at home if you are in a time crunch and can't make it to the gym on certain days.

SET UP A HOME GYM

If you prefer to set up a gym at home, you'll need to make sure you have the right equipment on hand to do the workouts properly. You'll need all of the equipment listed to the left except the cable system—you can use bands instead. You can find all of the below at www.performbetter.com.

→ Get a pair of dumbbells that weigh at least as much as your purse. They will likely be around 8 to 12 pounds. Then purchase the next two pairs up from that (for example, 15 and 20 pounds). Another great option is to get a set of Powerblocks, which give you a whole range of dumbbells to use but don't take up much space.

→ I recommend also getting one kettlebell that is about twice the weight of your purse.

→ Purchase three different strengths of bands. This will be your at-home cable system.

→ Purchase a TRX suspension trainer along with a door anchor, which you can find at www.trxtraining.com. This one piece of equipment will allow you to do many exercises.

→ A bench or a step. You may be able to use a stair step in your home, or a footstool. Make sure it is sturdy and can handle all of your body weight.

→ A yoga mat or a thick towel.

→ A foam roller, lacrosse ball, or The Stick.

→ It's also a good idea to devote an area of your home exclusively to exercising—whether it's in your garage, basement, or spare bedroom. If you live in a small apartment or have limited free space, consider purchasing a special basket or storage box that you can tuck under your bed or behind a couch when you're not working out.

Now you are ready to hit the gym—time to train!

The Workout Calendar

The following is the entire 12-week workout plan. Don't get overwhelmed! It's laid out here to make sure you can plan ahead and make time for all of the workouts, to achieve the best possible results. There's no need to second-guess or worry about which workouts to do—we've designed and honed this system to be effective. All you need to do is commit to taking it one day at a time.

If you miss a day or get off track, just pick up where you left off. Don't try to add or do extra. Simply do the workout you are supposed to do that day and get back on track. The plan calls for you to perform a strength workout every other day and one metabolic workout on Saturday. If this schedule doesn't fit with what works best for you, rearrange the days so it does.

RULES TO STICK TO:

→ *Do your best to take a day off between strength workouts. You can do two strength workouts back-to-back, if you have to, but never do three.*

→ *Make the strength workouts your priority. If you absolutely must miss a workout, miss the metabolic or the intervals.*

PHASE 1: Weeks 1-4

	Monday	Tuesday	Wednesday	Thursday	Friday	Saturday	Sunday
Week 1	**Day 1** STRENGTH WORKOUT 1	**Day 2** DAY OFF: Active Recovery	**Day 3** STRENGTH WORKOUT 2	**Day 4** DAY OFF: Active Recovery	**Day 5** STRENGTH WORKOUT 1	**Day 6** TIMED METABOLIC	**Day 7** DAY OFF: Active Recovery
Week 2	**Day 8** STRENGTH WORKOUT 2	**Day 9** DAY OFF: Active Recovery or optional 20-minute interval session	**Day 10** STRENGTH WORKOUT 1	**Day 11** DAY OFF: Active Recovery	**Day 12** STRENGTH WORKOUT 2	**Day 13** COUNT-DOWN METABOLIC	**Day 14** DAY OFF: Active Recovery
Week 3	**Day 15** STRENGTH WORKOUT 1	**Day 16** DAY OFF: Active Recovery or optional 20-minute interval session	**Day 17** STRENGTH WORKOUT 2	**Day 18** DAY OFF: Active Recovery	**Day 19** STRENGTH WORKOUT 1	**Day 20** TIMED METABOLIC	**Day 21** DAY OFF: Active Recovery
Week 4	**Day 22** STRENGTH WORKOUT 2	**Day 23** DAY OFF: Active Recovery or optional 20-minute interval session	**Day 24** STRENGTH WORKOUT 1	**Day 25** DAY OFF: Active Recovery	**Day 26** STRENGTH WORKOUT 2	**Day 27** COUNT-DOWN METABOLIC	**Day 28** DAY OFF: Active Recovery

PHASE 2: Weeks 5-8

	Monday	Tuesday	Wednesday	Thursday	Friday	Saturday	Sunday
Week 5	**Day** 29 STRENGTH WORKOUT 1	**Day** 30 DAY OFF: Active Recovery or optional 20-minute interval session	**Day** 31 STRENGTH WORKOUT 2	**Day** 32 DAY OFF: Active Recovery	**Day** 33 STRENGTH WORKOUT 1	**Day** 34 TIMED METABOLIC	**Day** 35 DAY OFF: Active Recovery
Week 6	**Day** 36 STRENGTH WORKOUT 2	**Day** 37 DAY OFF: Active Recovery or optional 20-minute interval session	**Day** 38 STRENGTH WORKOUT 1	**Day** 39 DAY OFF: Active Recovery	**Day** 40 STRENGTH WORKOUT 2	**Day** 41 COMPLEX METABOLIC	**Day** 42 DAY OFF: Active Recovery
Week 7	**Day** 43 STRENGTH WORKOUT 1	**Day** 44 DAY OFF: Active Recovery or optional 20-minute interval session	**Day** 45 STRENGTH WORKOUT 2	**Day** 46 DAY OFF: Active Recovery	**Day** 47 STRENGTH WORKOUT 1	**Day** 48 TIMED METABOLIC	**Day** 49 DAY OFF: Active Recovery
Week 8	**Day** 50 STRENGTH WORKOUT 2	**Day** 51 DAY OFF: Active Recovery or optional 20-minute interval session	**Day** 52 STRENGTH WORKOUT 1	**Day** 53 DAY OFF: Active Recovery	**Day** 54 STRENGTH WORKOUT 2	**Day** 55 COMPLEX METABOLIC	**Day** 56 DAY OFF: Active Recovery

PHASE 3: Weeks 9-12

	Monday	Tuesday	Wednesday	Thursday	Friday	Saturday	Sunday
Week 9	**Day** 57 STRENGTH WORKOUT 1	**Day** 58 DAY OFF: Active Recovery or optional 20-minute interval session	**Day** 59 STRENGTH WORKOUT 2	**Day** 60 DAY OFF: Active Recovery	**Day** 61 STRENGTH WORKOUT 1	**Day** 62 COUNT-DOWN METABOLIC	**Day** 63 DAY OFF: Active Recovery
Week 10	**Day** 64 STRENGTH WORKOUT 2	**Day** 65 DAY OFF: Active Recovery or optional 20-minute interval session	**Day** 66 STRENGTH WORKOUT 1	**Day** 67 DAY OFF: Active Recovery	**Day** 68 STRENGTH WORKOUT 2	**Day** 69 COMPLEX METABOLIC	**Day** 70 DAY OFF: Active Recovery
Week 11	**Day** 71 STRENGTH WORKOUT 1	**Day** 72 DAY OFF: Active Recovery or optional 20-minute interval session	**Day** 73 STRENGTH WORKOUT 2	**Day** 74 DAY OFF: Active Recovery	**Day** 75 STRENGTH WORKOUT 1	**Day** 76 COUNT-DOWN METABOLIC	**Day** 77 DAY OFF: Active Recovery
Week 12	**Day** 78 STRENGTH WORKOUT 2	**Day** 79 DAY OFF: Active Recovery or optional 20-minute interval session	**Day** 80 STRENGTH WORKOUT 1	**Day** 81 DAY OFF: Active Recovery	**Day** 82 STRENGTH WORKOUT 2	**Day** 83 COMPLEX METABOLIC	**Day** 84 DAY OFF: Active Recovery

Get Moving RAMP

This program includes a very specific warmup. Below, Craig Rasmussen explains why it is so important.

Most people who embark on an exercise regimen understand that they should do some type of warmup to start the session. But many people don't think it is all that important. If they're going to skip something in their workouts, the warmup is what they tend to skip. This is a mistake. Studies have shown that warming up and stretching improve physical performance and prevent injuries, especially a warmup that increases your body temperature and uses similar movements to the main workout activities. The Get Moving RAMP workout serves as your warmup and is extremely important. Don't skip it!

Traditional old-school warmups (such as walking on a treadmill or riding on an exercise bike) target the cardiovascular system and the lower body in only one plane of motion and in a very small range of motion. This does warm you up in one sense, but it is not nearly as productive as it could be, and it is pretty boring, to say the least. We can do much better! To properly prepare for an intense exercise session, we need to prepare the entire body in multiple planes of motion.

I prefer to not even call it a warmup. Instead, I call it RAMP, which stands for range of motion, activation, and movement preparation. This simple change in nomenclature immediately makes it sound more important (because it is!).

The Get Moving RAMP workout does several important things.

1. *Addresses soft tissue quality, like a massage does, to reduce any tension and/or knots (via the foam roller and the lacrosse ball)*

2. *Improves muscle length/extensibility*

3. *Improves mobility of the joints*

4. *Elevates body/core temperature and increases bloodflow*

5. *Takes the body through multiple planes of movement to improve mobility*

6. *Charges up and excites the nervous system to prepare the body for the demands of the workout and the movement patterns (exercises) that will follow. We need to prepare the body for the squat, bend, single leg stance, lunge, push, pull, and core movements.*

Every 4 weeks, you'll have brand-new Get Moving RAMP exercises to learn. This workout serves multiple purposes.

Your First Workout: Take yourself through these moves first before doing anything else. The goal is to get through them in 10 minutes. On Day 1, this may be all you do as you get moving. Each time you do it, though, you will feel less challenged and ready for more.

Your Warmup: Use this as your warmup throughout the 12-week program at the start of every strength workout and metabolic workout.

Your Recovery Workout: Throughout the 12 weeks, use the Get Moving RAMP exercises on your off days to regenerate and improve your recovery, get your blood flowing, work on range of motion and flexibility, and get moving without putting a training demand on your body.

Part of Your Strength Workout: You'll see four of these moves throughout your strength workouts, instead of resting: Hip Stretch/Mobilization, Hip Stabilizer Activation, Ankle Mobility, and Thoracic Spine Mobility. These four moves are a priority and will be done almost every day throughout the 12 weeks.

You'll really get to know all of the exercises in the RAMP workout because you'll do them almost every day, either as your warmup, as part of your workout, or as your recovery. You'll also see these exercises throughout your strength program—they fill in your rest periods and make the most effective use of your time. Use these Get Moving RAMP exercises to start every workout you do.

Some of the key areas that you'll need to focus on during these movements are the thoracic spine (upper back), the hips, and the ankles. These areas often tend to need increased mobility in most people. You'll also want to activate several key muscles such as the hip stabilizers (glutes) and the scapular stabilizers (small muscles around the shoulder blades).

The Get Moving RAMP workout contains the following:

Range of Motion: Stretching and/or mobility exercises.

Activation: Specific activation exercises for the often-dormant muscles around the hips and shoulder blades.

Movement Preparation: Dynamic stretching and movements that take the body through large excursions and multiple planes of motion.

A primary principle of "RAMPing" is that you start with exercises that are ground-based (done on or near the floor), done in place, and of fairly low intensity. You'll then progressively move to exercises that are done standing in place. Next, you'll start moving (locomotion), and the movements will become more dynamic in nature. As you can see, exercise intensity and exercise complexity gradually "ramp" up as you move through this period. This tends to make the RAMPing flow well and follow a logical sequence. It's like starting up a car in colder months and letting it warm up for a few minutes before you put it in gear, pull out, and drive it.

It should be noted that the order of the exercises can be changed a bit to follow the RAMPing principle that we discussed earlier—always starting on the ground, then standing, then moving. More than one exercise in a category can be added if needed, but the total amount of exercises should not exceed 8 to 12 (not including the foam roller/ball self-myofascial release).

The bottom line: Take your RAMP warmup seriously! It will better prepare you for the best training session possible, and it will help to keep your body healthier in the process.

RAMP Template

Each Get Moving RAMP workout has a minimum of 10 exercises plus foam rolling, all of which are there for a specific purpose. In Phase One you'll start by building a base strength. In Phases Two and Three you'll incorporate more dynamic movements into your warmup, to wake up your nervous system and improve your speed of movement.

1 Foam Roller/Ball SMR:
Each session starts with foam rolling and lacrosse ball self-massage (or self-myofascial release) to address soft tissue quality and help to iron out trigger points, knots, or adhesions.

2 Hip Stretch/Mobilization:
The hips are the centerpiece of the body and are an area of focus where we look to improve mobility. The first exercise is a stretch or mobilization for the hips (this can vary a bit depending on your needs, but will commonly be some sort of hip flexor stretch).

3 **Hip Stabilizer Activation Exercise (backside):** This will be some type of hip bridge to wake up the often-dormant gluteus maximus (butt) and develop motor control. Note that this is preceded by a stretch of the front side of the hips to better allow you to wake up your backside and take advantage of the new range of motion attained from the stretch.

4 **Hip Stabilizer Activation Exercise (side):** You'll move to an exercise such as a Side Lying Clam Shell to wake up the muscles on the outside of the hip, which help to control rotational and lateral movements of the upper leg. You'll want to turn up the "dimmer switch" on these muscles to wake them up as you prepare to integrate them into more complex movements.

5 **Thoracic Spine Mobility Exercise:** This movement improves the extension and rotation capabilities of the upper half of the spine. This is a problematic area in most people, and stiffness here can lead to a host of issues in the shoulders and lower back, so it is a major priority.

6 **Ankle Mobility Exercise:** This movement helps to improve dorsi-flexion, or the ability of the shin to move toward the foot. This is a critical component of several patterns including walking, running, sprinting, lunging, squatting, etc. Poor ankle mobility can be a component of knee pain as well.

7 **Scapular Stabilizer Activation Exercise:** Next up, you'll wake up the muscles that attach to your shoulder blades. We need to innervate some of the small stabilizer muscles such as the lower trapezius and the serratus anterior, which are often dormant and weakened muscles in the shoulder blades.

8 **Squat Mobility/Patterning Exercise:** You want to prepare your body for the demands of the squat pattern and integrate several of the key joints that you worked on earlier in the RAMP. Your goal is to develop a range of motion and control to enable you to squat deeply.

9 **Hip Separation Exercise (SL Stance):** This exercise will have you spend some time standing on one leg and working on flexing or rotating one of your hips while the hip on your opposite side is extended. You want to prepare your body for the demands of the single leg stance pattern.

10 **Sagittal Plane Lunge Exercise:** Next, you'll perform a lunge variation where your body moves in a more linear motion (straight ahead or straight back). Again, you're integrating several joints and "putting everything together." This prepares you for the lunge patterns that you'll use in resistance exercises.

11 **Frontal or Transverse Plane Lunge Exercise:** Finally, you'll perform another lunge variation that is performed to the side or with a rotational component of the hips. The hips require movement in multiple planes of motion, which is why they require several drills to properly address this need.

Strength Programs

The priority workouts in this plan focus on strength training. These are metabolically demanding, circuit-style routines that include all seven movements of the human body: squat, bend, push, pull, core stability, lunge, and single leg stance. You'll gain strength and hypertrophy (increase lean muscle size) while boosting your metabolism and burning fat. I know it sounds counterintuitive, but building muscle will help you shrink!

The strength workouts also include power and combination exercises along with core-strengthening exercises as priorities. You'll have two different, yet complementary, full-body routines per phase that you can alternate back and forth for 4 weeks. In each new phase you'll start all new routines to keep things fresh and fun.

Each workout has these components:

Core: For most women, this is one of the weakest areas, and specific core exercises need to be first in the program so that you can do them when you're the most fresh and energized. All of these exercises are about building core stability, which will help you master every other exercise in the program.

Power/Combination: For the first two phases, you'll perform a power exercise on Day 1 and a combination exercise on Day 2. Both of these are very athletic movements and are some of the most effective "bang for your buck" exercises.

Strength: The strength section of each workout includes all of the basic movements just mentioned, working your full body every time. With each new phase, the exercises will progress from the phase before. The reps (or number of times you perform the exercise) will also vary. This keeps your body "confused," so you don't fall into a rut and will continue to see results. You'll also recognize two exercises in each strength workout from the Get Moving RAMP, which are used during your rest period between strength exercises.

Finisher: At the very end of the workout, be prepared to dig deep and give everything you have left. You'll max out intensity to give your metabolism a final boost right at the end. Don't hold back! You got this.

Metabolic Programs

Welcome to your new cardio workout! The goal of these workouts is to get your heart pumping, rev up your metabolism, and work up a sweat in a short period of time. These workouts shouldn't take more than 30 minutes max, making them easy to do any time of day.

A 2011 review in the *Journal of Obesity* entitled "High-Intensity Intermittent Exercise and Fat Loss," author Stephen Boutcher, PhD, pointed out that the effect of regular aerobic exercise on body fat is negligible. In 2008, a study by the same author looked at the effects of high-intensity exercise versus steady-state, specifically with women, and found that after 15 weeks, only the high-intensity exercise group had a significant improvement in fat loss. There was a significant reduction in fat from their legs compared to their arms (usually a more stubborn spot for women).

I discussed these findings in detail in my first book, *The Female Body Breakthrough*. Since then, there continues to be evidence in support of ending the hours and hours spent on a treadmill and replacing them with shorter, metabolically demanding

Master the Movements

One of my goals when I designed these programs was for you to truly master the basic seven movements of the human body:

1. **Squat**
2. **Bend**
3. **Push**
4. **Pull**
5. **Core Stability**
6. **Lunge**
7. **Single Leg Stance**

You'll master all of them with these programs. Each movement can be practiced with a number of exercises. You'll notice that an exercise in your strength program in Phase One may show up in a later phase as a metabolic exercise. In addition, the metabolic workouts use many of the same movements more than once, which will help you become more familiar with them. Throughout the program, work on mastering each movement as you work out, and challenge yourself to get even stronger by adding additional weight.

workouts. High-intensity, intermittent exercise has been shown to be more effective at reducing body fat than any other type of exercise. It has also been shown to significantly increase both aerobic and anaerobic fitness, lower insulin resistance, and improve skeletal muscle fat oxidation and glucose tolerance. These workouts are short and intense, lasting from 6 seconds to 4 minutes per interval, with a rest period of about the same time.

You'll mix these up in four different ways: Timed, Countdown, Complex, and the optional 20-minute Interval Workout. You have the freedom to choose one of these four programs on your metabolic day or rotate through them as laid out in the plan.

Timed Metabolic Workouts: These workouts include five exercises that you will do in a specific amount of time. Push your intensity during the work period and then completely recover during the rest period before doing the next exercise. For example, you'll do five exercises three times, performing 15 sets in a row before taking a 2- to 3-minute rest. Using high-intensity circuit-style routines like this has been shown to be more effective at improving body composition than doing endurance or lower-intensity routines.

Countdown Metabolic Workouts: These are a favorite at my gym, but they're also one of the toughest workouts you'll do. You'll start with a certain number of repetitions on round one and perform four different exercises with that same number of reps, finishing with 20 to 40 seconds of hard sprinting or jumping rope. You'll then rest and repeat with fewer repetitions counting down. As you get more tired, you will do fewer repetitions, making it realistic to finish with the same intensity.

Complex Metabolic Workouts: These workouts enter the picture in Phase Two. By then you'll have learned the basic movements and built up a base strength. These workouts use dumbbells or a barbell heavy enough to get your heart pumping and create a metabolic disturbance, but light enough so you won't cause any tissue damage or need too much recovery. You'll perform 8 reps of each of four exercises in a row without stopping. This 2- to 3-minute set is your "interval." Rest for 90 seconds and repeat.

Optional 20-Minute Interval Workouts: If you have done three strength workouts and two metabolic workouts but you're itching to do more on a sixth day, tackle a short intense interval workout.

This can be done on a cardio machine such as a bike, stairmaster, or treadmill. Or get outside and run hill sprints, ride your bike, or climb stairs.

Active Recovery: At least 1 day a week you need to give your body a break! Let it rest and regenerate. You can go through the Get Moving RAMP workout two to three times to stretch and get your blood flowing, but otherwise, chill out and do something relaxing.

What I mean by "active recovery" is that just because it is your day off and you don't have a structured, planned workout, that doesn't mean you shouldn't continue living an active lifestyle. Do something you enjoy, such as going for a walk, enjoying a bike ride, taking a hike, or going golfing. If you have a hobby or have been meaning to revisit an old hobby, this is your time to do it! I love to take dance class twice a week as part of my active recovery.

The workouts in this plan are challenging and taxing, but that's why they are effective. Don't be afraid to dive in and give it your all! You'll soon feel stronger and more confident than ever.

Keep Your Body Wanting More

Give your body at least 1 day off a week, no matter what. You need at least 1 day to regenerate every week. In addition, if you feel like you need additional recovery every other week, take off an additional day. Many times your workouts will be of better quality if you do less, and you won't get burned out or start to feel exhausted. Don't sacrifice quality for quantity.

Take note of your progress: Are you able to do more each week? Lift more weight? Do more reps? You should be getting fitter if you take the time to recover. If not, do fewer workouts, but focus on your movements and perform the exercises thoughtfully and with precision. Many times less is more.

THE MENU PLANS

"The Drop Two Sizes program came along right when I needed it. It gave me the motivation to put my energy into more healthy pursuits. And you know what I discovered again? Exercise is the best medicine. Healthy body, healthy mind. I don't know what the future holds for me, but I know that when I'm taking care of myself, I'm better able to handle whatever life throws my way."

—MICHELE ROSETTE, DROPPED TWO SIZES IN 8 WEEKS

Let's talk a bit about what you need to get started in the kitchen. I'm certainly not asking you to go to culinary school, but it will be useful to learn some basic kitchen smarts and "tools" to get you on track to eating more healthfully and fueling your body with the right foods to complement your workout routines and help you slim down fast.

I am not a chef (or even close!). In fact, my husband teases me that I don't cook; I "heat things up." Okay, so I'm a fan of the idea that simple is better. I tend to rotate a few of my favorite dinners, like chicken stir-fried with mixed veggies, buffalo burgers with portobello mushrooms and spinach, and turkey chili. But I can follow a recipe and have been known to make a pretty mean shepherd's pie and pot roast, when I really want to impress. I've found that all you need are a few great, easy recipes to prepare a healthy, filling meal.

This is why I enlisted the help of Chris Mohr, PhD, RD, who has designed simple, delicious menus to give you (and me!) new ideas when it comes to creating healthy, tasty meals. (Believe it or not, I avoided tofu until I tried the Tofu Stir-Fry recipe on page 84.) Dr. Mohr developed a fitness challenge similar to the one laid out in this book and created these menus based on what worked with his clients—who also

Super Simple Pot Roast

I learned this recipe from Mike Roussell, PhD, and make it when I'm feeling extra domestic. Yum!

INGREDIENTS:

2 tablespoons extra virgin olive oil
2 pounds beef chuck shoulder roast
2 onions, chopped
2 cups chopped turnips
4 cups baby carrots
4 cloves garlic, minced
1 teaspoon salt
1 teaspoon pepper
1 tablespoon dried thyme
2 teaspoons dried rosemary
1½ cups beef broth (low sodium) or red wine

HOW TO PREPARE: Preheat the oven to 350°F. In a large ovenproof pot or Dutch oven over medium-high heat, heat 1 tablespoon of the olive oil. Add roast and brown on all sides. Remove roast from the pan and pour out liquid. Add the remaining 1 tablespoon olive oil, onions, turnips, carrots, and garlic. Cook until the onions begin to become translucent. Meanwhile, rub the roast with the salt, pepper, thyme, and rosemary on all sides. Add roast back to the pan along with the broth or wine. Cover tightly and simmer for 5 minutes. Place the pan in the oven and roast for 2½ to 3 hours, or until the roast can easily be pulled apart with a fork. Makes 5 servings.

ALTERNATIVE COOKING METHOD: Brown the roast and season it as directed above. Place in a slow cooker with the remaining ingredients and cook for 6 to 8 hours on low.

dropped two sizes in 12 weeks! Many of my clients have also used these recipes and gave them rave reviews.

GET TO KNOW YOUR KITCHEN

Sometimes the kitchen is so foreign that we stay away from it altogether and rely on unhealthy takeout or fast food. I had a client whose husband did 100 percent of the cooking. As she put it, "I only walked through the kitchen to get to another part of the house. I had no business even standing in there as I may have messed something up." They had very defined roles: Her husband worked and did the cooking, and she tended to the kids and maintained the house, as long as that didn't include food prep or cooking. One time, when their three kids were all under 10 years old, her husband had a meeting and was traveling out of town. He left my client a package of hot dogs, a box of mac and cheese, a pan, and a cookbook open to a page with a casserole recipe. It was pretty straightforward, or so he thought! "The kids ended up with very dry noodles that I had in the oven way too long," my client laughed. "So long, in fact, they wouldn't even touch the hot dogs. We ordered pizza that night."

You don't have to be intimidated by cooking, and you don't have to become Julia Child, either. These meal plans are really simple and designed for anyone to make and enjoy. The best part? They are tasty and effective at slimming you down.

All you really need to get started is a basic set of pots and pans. Nothing fancy. You can pick these up at any home goods store. You'll also want to have a decent set of cutlery (knives) as well. Food prep is significantly easier with sharp knives, and you'll actually run less of a risk of hurting yourself than with dull knives.

Other must-have items:

Blender (I like the Vitamix)
Can opener
Cutting board(s)
Colander
George Foreman Grill
Measuring cups
Measuring spoons

STOCK YOUR PANTRY

Now that you have your kitchen stocked with the basic tools, it's time to fill your pantry with the right ingredients. Once you've gotten the most basic spices and condiments, you can plan ahead each week to buy the foods you'll need for the weekly meal plans. I've already created a grocery list for you each week. To keep it simple, write down just the items you need from the meal plans to help you stay on track, and don't stray down the junk food aisle. Remember: If it's not in the house, you won't eat it! Using a targeted shopping list will help you be more successful.

If you can, choose one day each week when you have a little more time to go shopping, so you won't feel rushed and forget anything. If possible, try to shop alone—kids are sure to throw you off your game—and never shop hungry!

CUSTOMIZE YOUR MEALS

Because of the importance of protein, we've included a decent amount of fish, chicken, pork, and other sources of protein in this plan. Keep in mind that any protein sources work, so if you have a dietary restriction such as a fish allergy, feel free to substitute an equal amount of chicken or other source of protein. Don't like red meat? Not a problem—try a different protein like tofu or fish, for example.

We have also designed the recipes to be customizable to your taste—especially with the grilled items like chicken, pork, and red meat. We let you decide

Essential Seasonings & Condiments

Before you begin the 12-week meal plan, make sure you have the following seasonings and condiments on hand. You'll be using them frequently to create the delicious meals and snacks you'll be enjoying over the next 12 weeks. These can be found in any grocery store.

1. Black pepper
2. Kosher salt
3. Oregano
4. Basil
5. Crushed red-pepper flakes
6. Mrs. Dash (good on poultry, fish, and meat)
7. Chili powder
8. Ground cinnamon
9. Extra virgin olive oil
10. Canola oil
11. Sesame oil
12. Balsamic vinegar
13. Rice vinegar
14. Mayonnaise made with olive oil
15. Dijon mustard
16. Brown mustard
17. Low-sodium soy sauce
18. Honey or agave nectar
19. Cooking spray

what marinades or sauces to use, so you can control the flavors and find exactly what you like so you'll savor every bite. That said, here are a few seasoning suggestions.

Fish: lemon-pepper seasoning
  (Mrs. Dash makes one we like)
Pork and chicken: smoked paprika or chili
  powder with lime juice
Shrimp: lemon juice, salt, and pepper
Steak: a basic Montreal steak seasoning

SECRETS TO SUCCESS

Whatever helps you stick to the plan is a successful strategy for healthy eating! Below are some of the most popular tips and tricks I've culled from clients, as well as notes I've saved from my own journal entries.

CLEAN HOUSE. Get rid of any junk food or snacks that might be a trigger for you. If you need to keep certain foods around for your kids or husband that are not part of your plan, use a cupboard just for them that is off-limits to you. This is a strategy one of my clients uses with huge success. "The kids have their cupboard with their foods, and I don't ever go in there," she explains.

KEEP TRACK. Purchase a journal to use for this challenge to keep track of your nutrition and your workouts.

PLAN AHEAD. Don't make a big deal about it, don't stress about it, just do it! Each evening, think ahead to the next day and plan out what you're going to eat. You can use your journal to pencil in what you plan to eat during the next day or two. Stay calm and organized, and always make sure you have healthy food with you. Pack an insulated lunch bag every day so you're not tempted to stray from the plan. Remember that nothing tastes as good as lean and sexy feels!

COOK EXTRA PROTEIN. Any time you cook meat, poultry, fish, or other protein, make a little extra to keep on hand in your fridge to throw on a salad or just grab and go. Keep hard-cooked eggs in the fridge at all times for an easy snack. You can also keep cans of tuna and salmon at the ready as an easy source of protein.

COMMIT TO GETTING CREATIVE. Do whatever it takes to make dinners that keep you interested and excited. I use a fruit and vegetable delivery company that provides many different varieties of vegetables delivered to my home once a week.

I mix and match my produce with all kinds of protein options so I never get bored.

GET WILD IN THE FREEZER. Buy frozen wild-caught fish (orange roughy, cod, mahi mahi, tilapia, flounder) that can be cooked in just a few minutes for a quick meal. I've brushed Dijon mustard on a frozen salmon fillet, stuck it in the oven for 20 to 30 minutes, and served it with steamed veggies. Voilà—dinner is ready!

MAKE MRS. DASH YOUR FRIEND. I use this all-purpose seasoning on my dinner most nights, and many times on my eggs in the morning. It's a quick way to spice up a meal and keep my tastebuds happy. Salsa is also a figure-friendly condiment you can enjoy freely, and mustard works great as a dipping sauce for chicken or other protein.

SATISFY YOUR NEED FOR CRUNCH. Buy a small bag of coleslaw, rainbow slaw, or broccoli slaw and mix it with tuna, chicken, or other protein for an instantly satisfying, crunch-worthy salad. (Thanks, Dr. John Berardi!) I also sprinkle ground flax seeds on the salad for a nutty taste along with a little olive oil and balsamic vinegar. Keeping sliced cucumber or baby carrots in your fridge provides you with another good crunchy snack option.

My Grocery List

The following is most likely what you would see in my cart. I especially like to keep fresh fruits and veggies, Greek yogurt, and nuts and seeds on hand for easy, healthy snacks. I get most of my fruits and veggies from a company that delivers a weekly box of organic produce right to my home. This forces me to try new things, and I always have seasonal, organic food in the house.

1. Blueberries
2. Frozen berries
3. Small avocados
4. Eggs
5. Small cartons of egg whites
   (Sometimes these are just easier to scramble with some spinach.)
6. 2% Greek yogurt
7. Thin-sliced fresh chicken breast
8. Fresh fish (wild caught only)
9. Frozen fish
   (such as orange roughy, flounder, and cod)
10. Lean steak
11. Pork loin
12. Turkey burgers or ground turkey
13. Canned tuna or salmon in water
14. Canned coconut milk
    (Choose those whose only ingredients are coconut milk and water.)
15. Coffee
16. Green tea (I like Good Earth Tea.)
17. Sesame seeds
18. Slivered almonds

WHAT'S IN THIS PLAN

I'm always on the lookout for new information, a better or faster way to get effective results with my clients (and myself). When I come across something in research or reading, I try it myself first. Many times it stops there. If I feel like it might be appropriate, I'll have my staff try it out. (I have a few women on our team who love to be guinea pigs, trying new workouts and nutrition ideas—thanks, ladies!) If I still feel confident that it is in fact a better method, I'll introduce it to a few of my clients. This was how I developed the plan for my first book, and I've continued to hone my plan here.

Here are some of the key elements of this plan.

DAY-BY-DAY MENUS. Once you know the basic principles of the plan, you can choose the foods you like while still following those principles. However, many people still want a specific menu plan for every day, along with recipes. You're not required to follow these menus exactly for the 12 weeks, but they may help to give you ideas for new foods and recipes, how to prepare them, and what a successful day should look like on the plan.

AN OMEGA-3 AND VITAMIN D SUPPLEMENT. Omega-3 fish oils have been shown to increase fat oxidation, among other important health benefits. In addition, brand new research shows that adding fish oil supplements can help to build muscle and strength. Vitamin D has been proven in current and emerging research to be a mandatory supplement for health and vitality. Check out "Vitamin D: The Sunshine Vitamin" on page 49 for more on its important health benefits. Both are recommended on this plan.

TRUSTED BRANDS. When appropriate, I've listed specific brands on the grocery lists, such as Kashi Go Lean cereal and ak-mak or RyKrisp crackers. These products have good amounts of fiber and protein, but low sugar, plus the ingredients are all-natural. Many packaged products are highly processed, with high-fructose corn syrup listed as the first ingredient. By offering specific brands, I hope to make it easier for you to choose the right healthy snacks and other foods to satisfy your cravings!

A GREENS DRINK. Get your veggies in one easy serving! A greens drink should supplement an already very "green" diet—meaning one loaded with green and other colored fruits and veggies. Greens drinks are also a convenient way to consume enough vegetables on the go, when healthy eating is more difficult. They surely don't replace eating whole fruits and veggies, but they're a good way to get additional micronutrients, antioxidants, and phytochemicals. We like Greens+ and use it regularly on top of our clean diets. You can find Greens+ products at www.greensplus.com.

THE FUSS ABOUT FASTING

Since I wrote my last book, intermittent fasting has become the buzz, which goes against one of my rules, "Fuel Yourself to Be Fabulous." But, curiosity got the better of me, and I decided I couldn't knock fasting until I tried it. Does it work? Yes. Is it extreme? Yes. Is it necessary? Absolutely not.

Fasting is something I tried myself but never introduced to my team or my clients because it isn't realistic. A study done in London in 2011 of 107 women compared intermittent calorie restriction to continuous calorie restriction and found that they were equally effective for weight loss.

If the results are the same, I believe you are better off eating every day to have fuel

Boost Your Food Power

Your metabolism increases after you eat. This is especially true when you eat protein, which has the highest thermic effect of food. The thermic effect of food refers to the calories your body burns to process the food you eat. Studies have shown that a higher-protein diet, including increased dairy consumption as a protein source, promotes body fat loss. In addition, recent studies show that eating a protein and a fat together significantly increases metabolism more than eating protein with a low-fat meal. This plan is structured to encourage you to include protein and a fat at each meal, along with a fruit or vegetable, to take advantage of this extra metabolic boost.

for your workouts. A fueled body is sure to have a better workout, and quality workouts add up to more fat loss. When your body is fueled with clean foods (which we've laid out in the meal plans), you can lose fat, think clearly, process the right nutrients, and have energy for your workouts—all at the same time.

One thing I did learn from my fasting experiment was a new rule you'll hear more about on the road map, which is to de-emphasize dinner. You will survive if you don't have a big sit-down dinner and will get better results by front-loading your food intake earlier in the day. Also, if you miss a meal, it isn't the end of the world. Just beware of waiting too long and ending up in "The State of Total Star-vation," or you'll set yourself up to binge.

Overall, I recommend fueling your body with real food to be fabulous. It has worked for me and for my clients over and over again. Eating properly sets you up to be able to maintain your hottest body for the long-term. It's healthy and realistic, and it ensures your body has all of the nutrients it needs to thrive.

HOW TO USE THE PLAN

The first few days will be the hardest and most uncomfortable. You'll have moments where you'll want to default to your old habits. Commit to following the menus as closely as you can the first week, and be sure to plan ahead and get started on the right foot. Your mind needs to be strengthened just like your muscles. Each time you can say, "No, thank you" and don't cave to a craving, you are strengthening your mind and your body!

The first week, challenge yourself to get through the entire 7 days following the menus exactly to prove to yourself that you can. This will put you in situations where you will be forced to troubleshoot and come up with healthy strategies and habits right away no matter how crazy your day is. As the 12 weeks continue, you'll have the freedom to mix and match your meals, and splurge 10 percent each week, so you'll never feel deprived. Remember: There will always be another meal. And if you do end up splurging more than your 10 percent, all is not lost! You'll have Splurge Checks throughout your journey to make sure that on average you are hitting 10 percent.

Here are the general meal plan rules for the next 12 weeks:

1. *Eat breakfast as soon as possible in the morning, followed by a meal every 3 to 4 hours. Try to de-emphasize dinner and front-load your food intake earlier in the day. People who lose weight and keep it off tend to eat breakfast—it's a common habit you should adopt! Make breakfast your priority meal, not dinner.*

2. *Eat a high-quality protein source along with a healthy fat at every meal and snack.*

3. *Have an average of two servings of vegetables at each meal, working up to 10 servings a day.*

4. *Eat nonprocessed, natural, whole foods that only contain ingredients you can pronounce! The less processed the food, the better it is for your body.*

5. *Drink 64 ounces (eight glasses) of water each day.*

6. *Supplement with a multivitamin, 1 to 2 grams of an omega-3 supplement, and 1,000 IU of vitamin D daily.*

7. *Always support your workout with a recovery shake. You can drink this before, during, and/or after your workout session.*

8. *Stick to these rules 90 percent of the time, allowing yourself 10 percent to splurge. Update your journal daily to keep track of your progress.*

Vitamin D: The Sunshine Vitamin

Vitamin D has gotten a lot of attention lately, and for good reason. This "vitamin" (it's technically a hormone) has been shown to improve muscle strength as well as bone health, reduce type 1 and 2 diabetes, and help prevent cancer, Alzheimer's disease, arthritis, and a host of other ailments. A 2011 Canadian study also showed that women with higher dietary vitamin D intake have lower body fat.

Our bodies naturally make vitamin D from exposure to sunlight, but most people don't get outside enough, and when we do, we need to slather ourselves with sunscreen, which might hinder vitamin D production. We can get some vitamin D from foods, but the problem is that there aren't many appealing options—milk, wild-caught salmon, sardines, anchovies, egg yolks, and liver are the strongest sources. So what should we do?

It may be wise to add a vitamin D supplement to your diet. The recommended dose is 1,000 IU per day, unless your health-care provider tells you differently. A favorite product of ours is Nordic Naturals Ultimate Omega-D3, which also has a high concentration of omega-3s in addition to 1,000 IU of vitamin D—a true win-win!

PHASE ONE

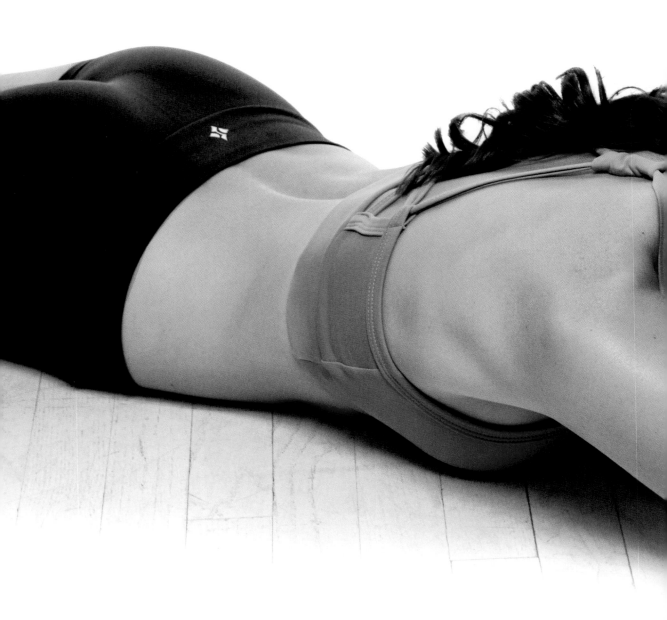

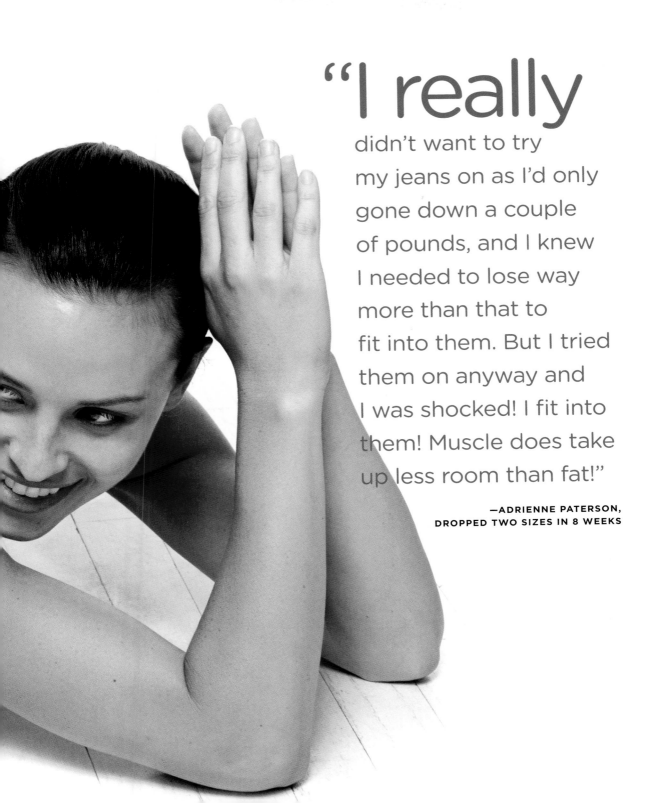

"I really

didn't want to try
my jeans on as I'd only
gone down a couple
of pounds, and I knew
I needed to lose way
more than that to
fit into them. But I tried
them on anyway and
I was shocked! I fit into
them! Muscle does take
up less room than fat!"

**—ADRIENNE PATERSON,
DROPPED TWO SIZES IN 8 WEEKS**

The first 30 days of this plan (or any plan!) are the most important. Most of my clients get hooked in the first 30 days, and the majority of them are successful. The ones who make their fitness goals a priority tend to be consistent and connect the positive results with the effort.

PHASE 1:
Road Maps

Read through the following weekly road maps before you get started, and then go through them again each week as you follow the plan. Commit to following the first 30 days of this plan as closely as possible. Get yourself hooked on feeling fit, rather than focusing on trying to reach a number on the scale by the end of the first month.

PHASE 1:
Meal Plan

The goal for the first 4 weeks is to eliminate the junk and start fueling your body with healthy, nutritious foods. Do your best to follow the menus as closely as you can, but if you need to swap or repeat a meal, it's fine.

We've provided specific foods with specific amounts, but you can exchange a protein for a protein, a vegetable for a vegetable, and so on. During this first phase, you can estimate the amounts and focus more on the quality of the foods you are eating, including more vegetables. Use these menus along with the road map to steer yourself in the right direction.

GOALS OF PHASE 1:

→ *Build healthy habits and strategies to set you up for success.*

→ *Eliminate the junk food and fuel your body with nutritious foods.*

→ *Learn how to plan ahead to avoid confusion and "The Lazy Cheat," page 113.*

→ *Get used to eating more vegetables. The goal for the first phase is to eat three servings of vegetables a day as a minimum.*

PHASE 1: **Workouts**

The following is your plan for the first 4 weeks. It's laid out here to make sure you can plan ahead and make time for all the workouts, to achieve the best possible results. Do not add anything, change anything, or skip anything. All you need to do is commit to taking it one day at a time!

	Monday	*Tuesday*	*Wednesday*	*Thursday*	*Friday*	*Saturday*	*Sunday*
Week **1**	**Day** 1 STRENGTH WORKOUT 1	**Day** 2 DAY OFF: Active Recovery	**Day** 3 STRENGTH WORKOUT 2	**Day** 4 DAY OFF: Active Recovery	**Day** 5 STRENGTH WORKOUT 1	**Day** 6 COUNT-DOWN METABOLIC	**Day** 7 DAY OFF: Active Recovery
Week **2**	**Day** 8 STRENGTH WORKOUT 2	**Day** 9 DAY OFF: Active Recovery or optional 20-minute interval session	**Day** 10 STRENGTH WORKOUT 1	**Day** 11 DAY OFF: Active Recovery	**Day** 12 STRENGTH WORKOUT 2	**Day** 13 COMPLEX METABOLIC	**Day** 14 DAY OFF: Active Recovery
Week **3**	**Day** 15 STRENGTH WORKOUT 1	**Day** 16 DAY OFF: Active Recovery or optional 20-minute interval session	**Day** 17 STRENGTH WORKOUT 2	**Day** 18 DAY OFF: Active Recovery	**Day** 19 STRENGTH WORKOUT 1	**Day** 20 COUNT-DOWN METABOLIC	**Day** 21 DAY OFF: Active Recovery
Week **4**	**Day** 22 STRENGTH WORKOUT 2	**Day** 23 DAY OFF: Active Recovery or optional 20-minute interval session	**Day** 24 STRENGTH WORKOUT 1	**Day** 25 DAY OFF: Active Recovery	**Day** 26 STRENGTH WORKOUT 2	**Day** 27 COMPLEX METABOLIC	**Day** 28 DAY OFF: Active Recovery

PHASE 1:
RAMP

Perform one set of each of the following warmup exercises before you start each workout.

1 **Foam Roller/Self-Myofascial Release Full Body**

2 **Half-Kneeling Hip Flexor Stretch with Rotation**
(8-10 reps with a 30-second hold on each side)

3 **Double Leg Hip Bridge**
(8–10 reps, holding for 5 seconds at the top of each rep)

4 **Side Lying Clam Shell**
(8–10 reps on each side with a 2-second hold at the top of the movement)

5 **Heel Sit Quadruped T-Spine with External Rotation** (8–10 reps on each side)

6 **Squat to Stretch** (8–10 reps)

7 **Wall Slide** (8–10 reps)

8 **Wall Standing Ankle Mobility**
(8–10 reps on each side)

9 **Wall Knee Marching** (5 reps on each side)

10 **Alternating Stationary Lateral Squat**
(5 reps on each side)

11 **Reverse Lunge with Overhead Reach**
(5 reps on each side)

RAMP 1:
Foam Roller/ Self-Myofascial Release

Before you go through the Get Moving RAMP workout, use a foam roller or a ball (a lacrosse or tennis ball works) to massage any areas that feel tight. These tools work to massage your muscles without having to spend big bucks for a professional masseuse.

Start with the six foam rolling exercises shown here. Your muscles will probably be tender the first time you roll them out, but don't push through any pain. You'll end up more tense, and it won't be effective. Each time you use the foam roller it will feel less uncomfortable.

Experiment rolling other areas that might be tight, such as the side of your leg (lie on your side and roll from your hip to just above your knee); your adductors (lie on your stomach, place the roller just above the inside of your knee and roll up to your inner thigh); and your chest (place a ball between your chest and a wall, just inside the front of the shoulder blade and below the collar bone, and roll back and forth).

Ideally, use the foam roller a few minutes each day to avoid injury and feel great after your workouts!

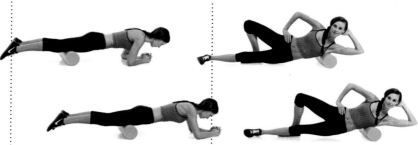

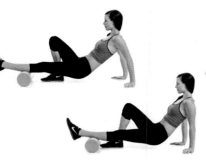

Calves

POSITION: Place your left calf on the roller and support yourself, putting as much weight on the calf as you can. Turn your left leg in and roll so you are massaging the inside of your left calf. Then turn your toe straight up and roll and finish with your toe turned out. Repeat on the opposite leg.

Quads

POSITION: Roll right over so the roller is on the tops of the fronts of your legs and lean to one side. Roll up and down and then switch to the other side.

Lats

POSITION: Lie on the roller so that it is under your armpit, and roll from your armpit to your hip along your lat with your bottom arm extended or bent behind your head.

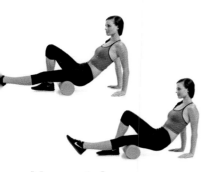

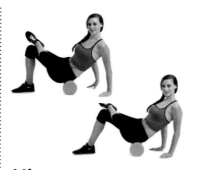

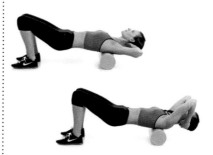

Hamstrings

POSITION: With your leg straight out and your hands behind you with your weight back on your arms, roll from the top of your leg where your hamstring goes into your hip right down to your knee. Put your weight on one leg and roll up and down, and then massage the other leg.

Hips

POSITION: Sit on the foam roller, cross your left leg over your right, and lean toward your left hip, putting your weight on your left hand. Roll on your glute and stop if you feel a spot that feels like a knot. Switch sides.

Thoracic Mobilization

POSITION: With the foam roller across your upper back, place your hands behind your head to support your neck. With your elbows up and out, roll slowly up and down your upper back as you extend and relax back onto the roller.

RAMP 2: Half-Kneeling Hip Flexor Stretch with Rotation

You will use the half-kneeling position frequently throughout your workouts for stretches, strength exercises, and core exercises. Practice this position, getting used to it, before you go into the hip flexor stretch and rotation.

START: Begin with your left knee on the floor (with a towel under it for padding, if you prefer) and your right leg lunged in front of you with your foot flat on the floor, as if you are in a "Will you marry me?" pose.

MOVEMENT: Place your hands behind your head with your elbows opened out. Squeeze your left butt cheek as you stretch the front of your left hip in a small range of motion to keep your hips underneath you and come back to the start. After performing all of your repetitions, repeat on the other side.

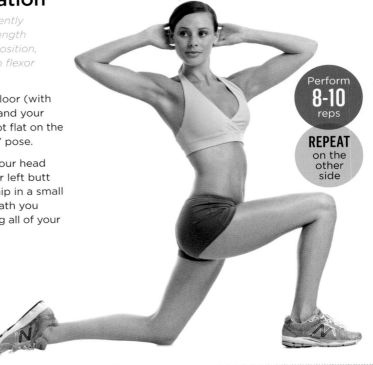

Perform
8-10
reps

REPEAT
on the other side

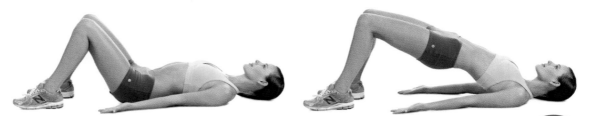

RAMP 3: Double Leg Hip Bridge

This exercise switches on your glutes, engages your core, and gives you an active stretch for the hip flexors. You'll also see it in your strength program as your active rest.

Perform
8-10
reps

START: Lie on your back with your knees bent and feet flat on the floor. Your arms should be out straight with your palms facing up.

MOVEMENT: Squeeze your glutes and lift your hips off the floor until your knees, hips, and shoulders are in one straight line, engaging your core and your glutes. Hold for 5 seconds and then lower back to the floor.

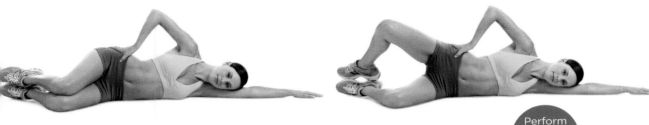

RAMP 4: Side Lying Clam Shell

This exercise works the external rotators of the hip to strengthen and improve range of motion. You'll feel your outer thigh and hip burning. This is really great for warming up your hips and may remind you of an old-school Jane Fonda move where you "feel the burn."

Perform **8-10** reps

REPEAT on the other side

START: Lie on your left side with your knees bent at a 90-degree angle, hips at a 45-degree angle, and your head resting on your left arm. Place your right thumb on your right hip bone and wrap your fingers around your hip to keep your hips still.

MOVEMENT: Lift your right knee off your left knee by externally rotating at the hip while keeping your pelvis still. Only lift your knee as high as you can without twisting your upper body and pelvis. Hold for 2 seconds. Lower your knee back down. Complete all of your reps and then switch sides.

RAMP 5: Heel Sit Quadruped T-Spine with External Rotation

Most people spend the majority of their days hunched over their desks, in their cars, on the phone, or on their laptops. This move is extremely important to get your upper back moving after being rounded over all day.

START: Get down on all fours. With your toes tucked under, sit back on your heels and place your right hand on the back of your head, your left forearm on the floor in front of your knees.

MOVEMENT: Rotate your right elbow up toward the ceiling, opening up your chest. Perform all of your reps and then repeat on the other side.

Perform **8-10** reps

REPEAT on the other side

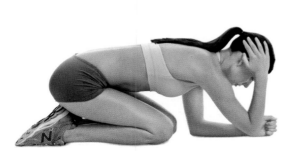

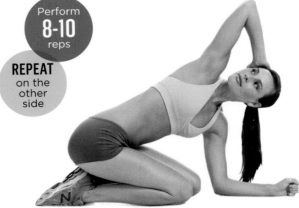

RAMP 6: Squat to Stretch

Take your time with this one and really sit into the squat and stretch and then straighten your legs for a good hamstring stretch. Each time you should get a little deeper in the stretch.

START: Assume a squat stance with your feet about shoulder-width apart and toes very slightly flared outward. Grasp your toes.

MOVEMENT: Bend forward at your hips so that your weight shifts to your heels. Next, keep your arms straight and inside your knees as you pull your rear end down and squat as low as you can. Lift your chest at the bottom of the movement. While still holding on to your toes, bring your rear end back up, stretching the back side of your body. Repeat. You will grasp your toes for the duration of the movement.

Perform **8-10** reps

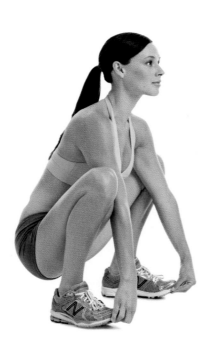
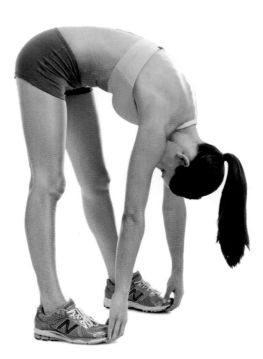

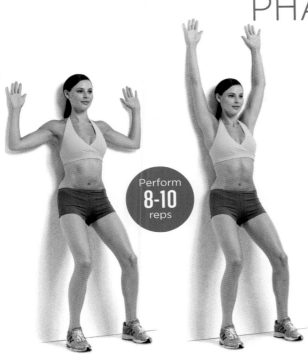

Perform **8-10** reps

RAMP 7: Wall Slide

This exercise will open up your chest and shoulders, getting you into good posture, warming up your shoulders, and improving your range of motion.

START: Stand with your back against a wall, with your head, upper back, and butt all touching the wall and your lower back in a neutral position. Place the back of your hands and arms against the wall.

MOVEMENT: Keeping your lower back from arching off the wall, slide your hands, arms, and elbows up the wall, keeping all three in contact with the wall. Reach as high as you can while maintaining contact. Then slide back down.

OPTION: *Perform this exercise using your TRX for resistance instead of the wall.*

RAMP 8: Wall Standing Ankle Mobility

If high heels are a part of your wardrobe, you probably have really tight ankles. Perform this ankle mobility exercise to undo some of the damage high heels create. I'm not saying don't wear them, I'm just saying do this exercise! It is so important that you'll be doing it in the warmup and in the strength workout.

START: Face a wall in a split stance with your front foot a couple of inches away from the wall. Place your hands on the wall to balance yourself.

MOVEMENT: While keeping the heel of your front foot down, bend your front knee toward the wall. Focus on keeping the knee tracking over your pinkie toe. You should feel a stretch in your Achilles, ankle, and/or calf muscle. Complete all of your reps and then switch legs.

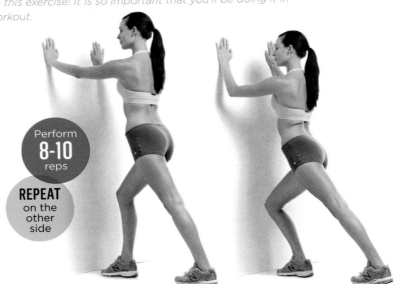

Perform **8-10** reps

REPEAT on the other side

RAMP 9: **Wall Knee Marching**

The goal is to be able to move your lower body and upper body while engaging your core. This exercise focuses on just that. Keep your core engaged as you work on the range of motion at each hip as you balance on one leg and then the other.

START: Face a wall with both hands flat against the wall at shoulder height. Walk your feet two steps away from the wall so that you are leaning into the wall. Your hips should be in line with your shoulders and your ankles.

MOVEMENT: Drive your left knee up as you drive up onto your right toes with your core engaged and the glute of the right leg engaged. Lower and alternate sides.

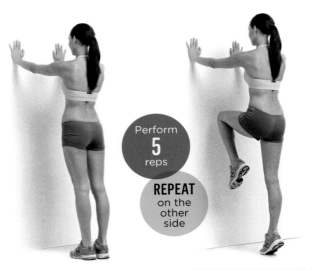

Perform **5** reps

REPEAT on the other side

RAMP 10: **Alternating Stationary Lateral Squat**

You'll be doing weighted lateral lunges in the strength program, so take your time with this exercise to warm up and stretch your inner thighs so you'll be ready for your workout.

START: Stand with your feet wider than shoulder-width apart. Place your arms straight out in front of you to offset your balance and keep your spine straight during the movement.

MOVEMENT: Keeping your feet stationary, shift your weight as you lunge to your right leg, sitting your hips back while keeping your right knee tracking over your right toes and stretching out your left inner thigh. Go only as low as you are comfortable with. Return to the center. Alternate sides.

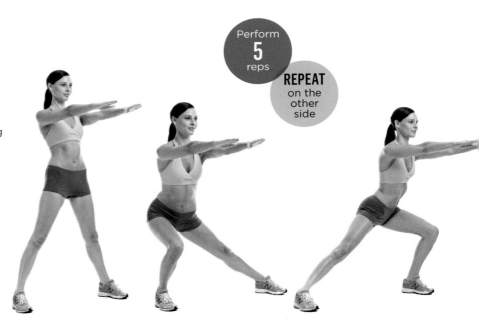

Perform **5** reps

REPEAT on the other side

RAMP 11: **Reverse Lunge with Overhead Reach**

You'll finish your warmup and get your entire body ready from head to toe with this lunging exercise. In Phase Two, you'll see this as part of your metabolic workout. After this, you should be ready to tackle your workout, or if you're just going through the Get Moving RAMP workout, then use this as your final movement. Be sure to really think about keeping your core engaged while using the front leg to drive up from the lunge.

START: Stand with your feet shoulder-width apart.

MOVEMENT: Looking straight ahead, step back into a lunge with your right leg as you reach both arms overhead. Your toes should stay straight forward, your front knee should be over your ankle and tracking over your toes, and your core should be engaged with good posture. Return to the start position and repeat with your left leg.

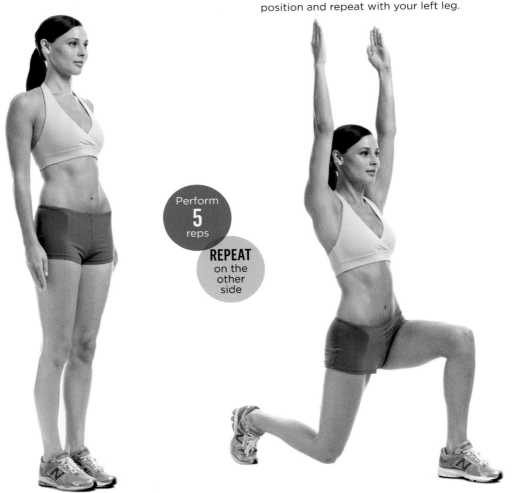

Perform
5
reps

REPEAT
on the
other
side

PHASE 1: Strength
Workout 1

Remember to do the Get Moving RAMP exercises to warm up! Then perform the following exercises as described in the chart.

Exercise	Sets	Reps	Speed	Rest
CORE				
1A **Plank with Alternating Leg Lift**	1-2	8 each side	Mod	None
1B **Alternating T-Stabilization**	1-2	8 each side	Mod	45 secs
POWER				
2 **High Pull**	1-2	10	Fast	1 min
STRENGTH				
3A **Goblet Squat**	2-3	15	Slow	1 min
3B **Three-Point Dumbbell Row**	2-3	15 each side	Slow	None
3C **Wall Standing Ankle Mobility**	2-3	10 each side	Mod	None
4A **Lateral Lunge with Contra Load**	2-3	15 each side	Slow	1 min
4B **Half-Kneeling Single Arm Overhead Press**	2-3	15 each side	Slow	None
4C **Wall Slide**	2-3	10	Mod	None
FINISHER				
5 **Body Weight Speed Squat**	2-4	20 secs	Fast	20 secs

1A Plank with Alternating Leg Lift

The goal is to stabilize your core (that is, don't move from your hips to your shoulders) while lifting one leg and then the other. Doing this exercise properly will strengthen your abdominals and back while also switching on your butt. This combination is guaranteed to improve the look of your stomach and your buttocks.

Perform **8** reps

REPEAT on the other side

START: Get in a plank position with your elbows on the floor directly underneath your shoulders, your back in a straight line, and your abdominal muscles braced.

MOVEMENT: While maintaining a neutral spine and tight abdominals and keeping your body as still as you can, lift your right leg up only 3 to 6 inches while engaging your glutes. Return to the starting position and then repeat with your left leg.

OPTION: *If this movement is difficult, perform it on an incline, resting your upper body on a sturdy object to decrease the load on your core.*

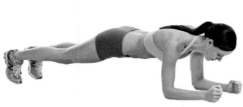

1B Alternating T-Stabilization

Rotational movements are so important when it comes to your workouts. This will fire your core, engage your shoulders, and get your whole body working as one unit.

START: Get in a pushup position with your head, upper back, and hips in a straight line.

MOVEMENT: Shift your weight and turn your hips and shoulders square to the wall, shifting your weight onto your bottom arm and bottom foot as you reach your free hand up toward the ceiling, forming a T. Keep your body in a straight line and shift back to the start position. Repeat on the other side, alternating back and forth.

Perform **8** reps

REPEAT on the other side

OPTION: *If this movement is difficult, perform it on an incline, resting your upper body on a sturdy object to decrease the load on your core.*

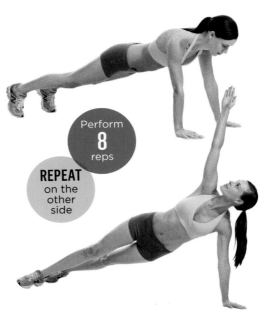

Perform
10
reps

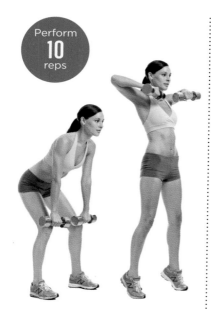

2 High Pull

This is the first power exercise you'll do, and you'll see it later as part of a combination and as part of your metabolic workout. The key is to use the power from your legs and hips to explode the weights up without muscling them up.

START: Hold a dumbbell in each hand or a barbell across your front.

MOVEMENT: Bend your knees and hips as if you're going to jump, sticking your hips back. From this position, explode into an extension with your hips, knees, and ankles. The momentum should propel the dumbbells or barbell up, with your elbows high and the dumbbells or barbell staying in close to your body, reaching chest height. Lower back down immediately and repeat.

3A Goblet Squat

Squats are one of the core exercises of this program because they work pretty much everything, burn a ton of calories, and challenge your body. The Goblet Squat is an excellent exercise because you cannot cheat. With a back squat most women will have a tendency to round their backs and lose their form. During a Goblet Squat, you have to keep your posture upright, holding the dumbbell or barbell using your upper back to support the load.

START: Stand with your feet shoulder-width apart, with your feet either straight or slightly rotated out. With both hands, hold a dumbbell in close to your chest with your elbows underneath it, supporting the weight.

MOVEMENT: Squat as deeply as you can without letting your back round over. Think about keeping your chest up and your knees tracking over your toes. As you come up, watch that you keep your knees from collapsing in.

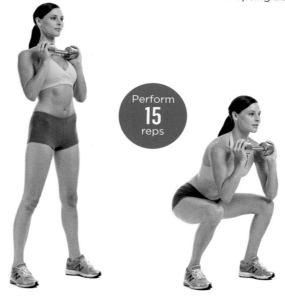

Perform
15
reps

OPTION: *If you're having trouble with the squat movement, you can use your TRX to hold onto and de-load this exercise, making it easier as you get stronger, rather than holding a weight.*

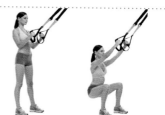

3B Three-Point Dumbbell Row

You can't just work what you see in the mirror—your back is what holds your posture upright and makes you look good as you walk out of the room too. As you perform this exercise, really engage the muscles in your back to build a nice sculpted upper back.

START: Stand in front of a bench with your feet shoulder-width apart. Bend over and support yourself by placing your left hand on the bench while holding a dumbbell in your right hand. Your feet should be directly under your hips, and your back should be flat with your head, spine, and tailbone in a straight line. The dumbbell should be hanging straight down from your right arm.

MOVEMENT: Row the dumbbell up by squeezing your shoulder blade back while maintaining a neutral spine. Lower the dumbbell and repeat. Do not shrug your shoulder; the movement should all be from your back. Repeat with your left arm.

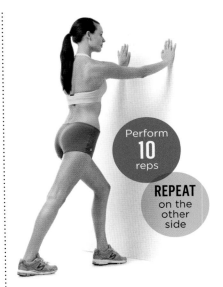

Perform **10** reps

REPEAT on the other side

Perform **15** reps

REPEAT on the other side

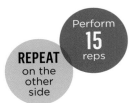

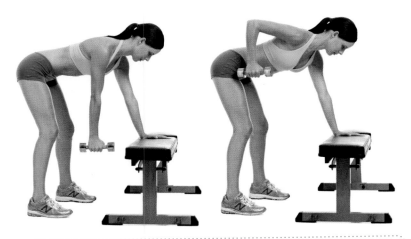

WHY THREE POINTS? *This exercise is called Three-Point Dumbbell Row because you are supported by your arm and both legs. You'll progress to a Two-Point Dumbbell Row that will work to further stabilize your core.*

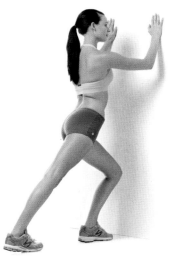

3C Wall Standing Ankle Mobility

Perform as described on page 59. Good ankle mobility means you can move better, which means you burn more calories!

4A Lateral Lunge with Contra Load

Forget the inner thigh machine. After performing this exercise, your inner thighs will be sore tomorrow. Really work on your range of motion while keeping your spine straight.

START: Stand with your feet shoulder-width apart and hold a kettlebell or dumbbell in your right hand. Your shoulders should be back with good posture.

MOVEMENT: Take a wide step out with your left leg laterally as you bend your knee and lunge, sitting back with your hips, and touch the weight to the inside of your left foot. Maintain a neutral posture with your lower back. Drive off your left leg and return to the start position. Repeat on the same side for 15 reps. Then switch sides.

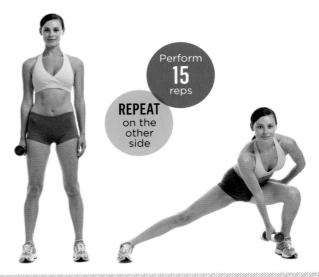

Perform
15
reps

REPEAT
on the other side

4B Half-Kneeling Single Arm Overhead Press

Perform
15
reps

REPEAT
on the other side

You will use this half-kneeling position often. Practice really bracing yourself by squeezing your glutes and stabilizing your core.

START: Get in a half-kneeling position with your right knee on the floor and your left knee up, and hold a single dumbbell at shoulder height with your right hand. Engage your glutes and core to keep your hips, knees, and shoulders in line and your upper-body posture upright.

MOVEMENT: Keeping your body still, push the dumbbell overhead, extending your arm all the way up. Be careful not to lean your body as you are pressing the dumbbell up. Lower the dumbbell back to the start position and repeat. Then switch sides.

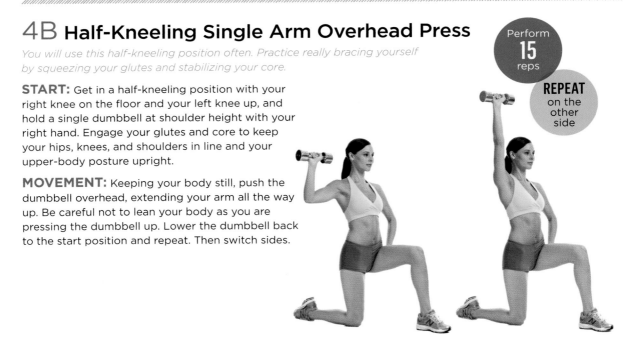

4C Wall Slide

Perform as described on page 59. This is a great movement to do during a Posture Check. You will open up your chest and shoulders.

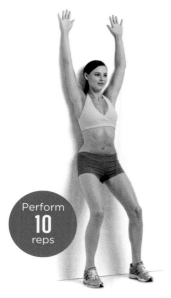

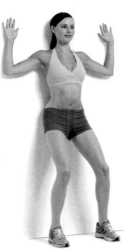

Perform
10
reps

5 Body Weight Speed Squat

Use the same form you used during your Goblet Squats with your back upright and your knees tracking over your toes. Do not let your heels pop up. The difference is that you are doing it with your body weight only this time.

START: Stand tall with your feet shoulder-width apart. Fold your arms behind your head, with your elbows out.

MOVEMENT: Squat until your thighs are parallel or below to the floor, return to the start position, and repeat. Keep your knees tracking over your toes, and keep your heels down the entire time.

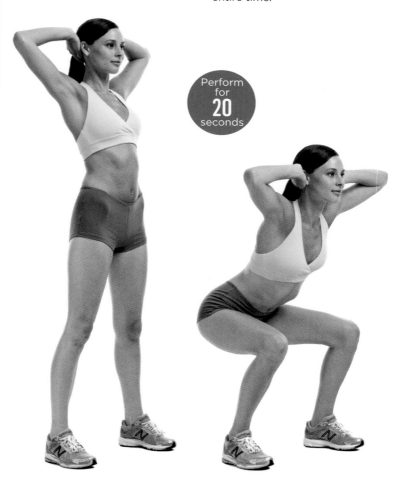

Perform
for
20
seconds

PHASE 1: Strength
Workout 2

Remember to do the
Get Moving RAMP exercises
to warm up! Then perform
the following exercises
as described in the chart.

Exercise	Sets	Reps	Speed	Rest
CORE				
1A **Side Plank with Rotation**	1-2	8 each side	Mod	None
1B **Active Leg Lowering**	1-2	8 each side	Mod	45 secs
COMBINATION				
2 **Reverse Lunge with Cable Row**	1-2	10 each side	Fast	1 min
STRENGTH				
3A **Romanian Deadlift**	2-3	15	Slow	1 min
3B **Pushup**	2-3	15	Slow	None
3C **Hip Flexor Stretch with Rotation**	2-3	30 sec each side	Hold	None
4A **Stepup**	2-3	15 each side	Slow	1 min
4B **Pulldown**	2-3	15	Slow	None
4C **Double Leg Hip Bridge**	2-3	10	Slow	None
FINISHER				
5 **Mountain Climber**	2-4	20 secs	Fast	20 secs

1A Side Plank with Rotation

Rotational core stabilization is also important, which is why this exercise is in the mix.

START: Lie on your side with your bottom elbow directly underneath your shoulder and your shoulders and feet stacked on top of each other, your back in a straight line, and your abdominal muscles drawn in tightly. Lift your hips off the ground, putting your weight on the forearm of your bottom arm and the side of your bottom foot. Your body should be in one straight line. Reach your top arm up toward the ceiling.

MOVEMENT: While maintaining the side plank position, take the top arm that is reaching toward the ceiling and bring it around your body and slide your hand under your body as if to stick your hand in your pocket. Then reach it back up to the ceiling.

OPTION: *If this exercise is difficult, perform it on an incline, resting your upper body on a sturdy object to decrease the load on your core.*

1B Active Leg Lowering

This exercise is all about working the deep underlying abdominal muscles that many women have forgotten how to engage. If you're doing it correctly, you will feel it.

START: Lie on your back with your legs pointing up to the ceiling. Think about keeping your ribs down, pulling your belly button toward the floor through your back. Pretend you're holding in your urine (yes, like Kegel exercises). Place your fingers just inside your hip bones to feel the deep muscle contracting.

MOVEMENT: While keeping your core stable completely, lower your right leg until it's just barely off the floor, hold for a count of 2 seconds, and then return to the start position. Repeat with your left leg. During each rep, really focus on keeping your core tight and engaged while moving your leg slowly and controlled.

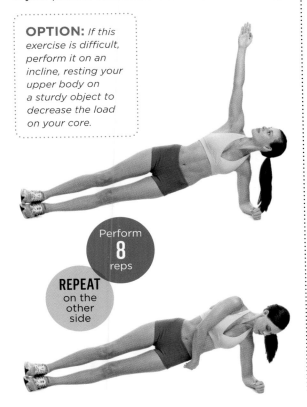

Perform
8
reps

REPEAT
on the
other
side

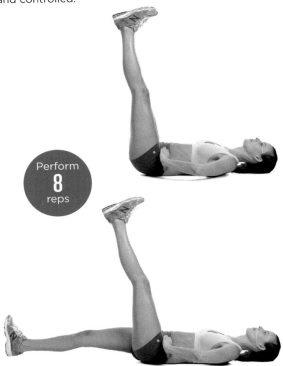

Perform
8
reps

2 Reverse Lunge with Cable Row

Throughout the program you'll see combination moves, which give you the most bang for your buck when it comes to an exercise. With this one we are getting the benefits of a row and a lunge; pairing them up equals a big-time calorie burn.

Perform
10
reps

REPEAT
on the
other
side

START: Grasp a cable with your right hand. Stand up tall with your feet shoulder-width apart, chest up, shoulders back, head looking straight ahead, and core tight.

MOVEMENT: Keeping your upper body still, shift your weight to one foot and lift the opposite foot behind you, engaging your glute to lift the leg and step back about 2½ feet as you lower your back knee to the floor into a lunge position. Driving through your front leg, return to the start position as you perform a row.

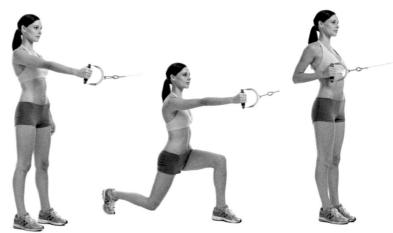

3A Romanian Deadlift

This exercise usually hits you the next day. While you're doing it, you won't feel like it's too challenging, but the next day you'll know you did it because the back of your legs and your butt will be sore. Really work on getting your form correct.

Perform
15
reps

START: Stand with your feet shoulder-width apart and hold dumbbells or a barbell in front of you, resting on your thighs.

MOVEMENT: Kicking your hips back and keeping the weight right along your legs, lower until you feel a stretch in your hamstrings, but be sure to maintain a neutral spine. Do not round your back. Keep your knees slightly bent, not locked, as you push your hips back. Return to the start position.

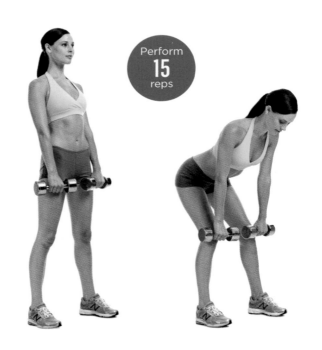

3B Pushup

For most women, the weak link on a pushup is the core. There are many different ways you can do a pushup to make it harder or easier. You can do it on an incline, using TRX straps, or, if necessary, on your knees on the floor. You can also perform a plank to pushup movement, working on your core strength first before you add the actual pushup.

START: Get in a pushup position on the floor, on an incline using a bench, or against a wall to support yourself, depending on how strong you are. If you are strong enough, do traditional pushups on the floor. Otherwise, the higher the incline, the easier this will be. Your spine should be in a straight line with your head, upper back, and tailbone in alignment.

MOVEMENT: Lower yourself until your shoulders go just below your elbows and then return to the start position, keeping your body in a straight line and your abdominals tight during the entire movement. If you cannot get the full range of motion without letting your back arch or without sticking your hips out, either increase the incline, perform a plank to pushup, or do the pushup on your knees.

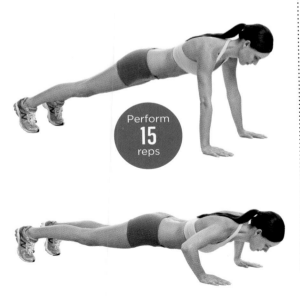

Perform
15
reps

3C Hip Flexor Stretch with Rotation

You will use the half-kneeling position frequently throughout your workouts for stretches, strength exercises, and core exercises. Practice this position before you go into the Hip Flexor Stretch with Rotation.

START: Begin with your left knee on the floor (with a towel under it for padding, if preferred) and your right leg lunged in front of you with your foot flat on the floor, as if you are in a "Will you marry me?" pose.

MOVEMENT: Place your hands behind your head with your elbows opened out. Squeeze your left butt cheek as you stretch the front of your left hip in a small range of motion to keep your hips underneath you and come back to the start. After performing all of your repetitions, repeat on the other side.

Perform
10
reps

REPEAT
on the other side

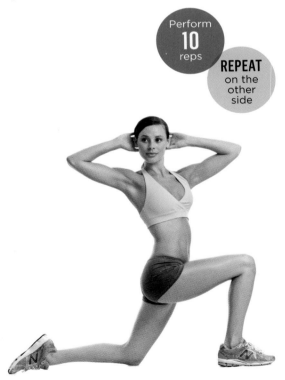

4A Stepup

The stepup is one of my all-time-favorite butt and leg exercises. The higher the step you use, the more your butt will be working in a full range of motion. Just don't go so high that you have to push off your bottom leg to drive yourself up.

START: Hold a dumbbell in each hand. Standing in front of a step, place your left foot on the step with your posture upright.

MOVEMENT: Shift your weight onto your left foot and drive your body up onto the step. Do not put your weight on your right foot. Lower yourself slowly back down to the start position and repeat for 15 reps. Then switch sides. Be careful you don't bounce off your bottom leg too much; instead try to really drive through the heel of your top leg to pull yourself up.

Perform **15** reps

REPEAT on the other side

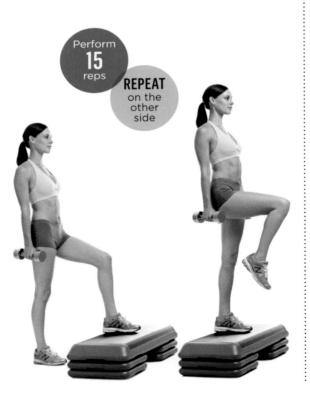

4B Pulldown

As a woman, you may have been told that you'll never do a pullup. Nonsense. Start with a pulldown movement, and as you're performing this movement, visualize that one day you will perform a pullup.

START: If you can perform the pulldown in a kneeling position, sit tall on your knees with a band or a pulley coming from above. Hold the handles of the pulley with your arms extended. Your hips should be directly over your knees and under your shoulders so that your ears, shoulders, hips, and knees are in a straight line. Otherwise, you can use a seated pulldown machine if an overhead pulley is not available to kneel under. Take an underhand grip with your palms facing you about shoulder-width apart, either on handles or on a bar.

MOVEMENT: Pull the weight down by bending your elbows, bringing them toward your body and your chest up toward the bar or handles. Keep your shoulders down as you pull down, and think about pulling your shoulder blades down and back. Finish with your arms against your body, elbows bent. Slowly extend back to the start position. Repeat for 15 reps.

Perform **15** reps

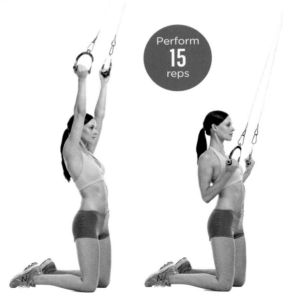

4C Double Leg Hip Bridge

This exercise switches on your glutes, engages your core, and gives you an active stretch for the hip flexors. You'll also see it in your strength program as your active rest.

START: Lie on your back with your knees bent and feet flat on the floor. Your arms should be out straight with your palms facing up.

MOVEMENT: Squeeze your glutes and lift your hips off the floor until your knees, hips, and shoulders are in one straight line, engaging your core and your glutes. Hold for 5 seconds and then lower back to the floor.

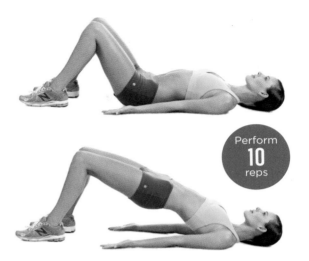

Perform
10
reps

5 Mountain Climber

For this exercise, you can use your body weight only, and if you need to, you can also do these on an incline either against a bench or using a TRX. Keep your body in a straight line and your core engaged as you drive your knees up one at a time.

START: Assume a standard pushup position with your head, shoulders, and butt in a straight line.

MOVEMENT: Drive one knee up toward your chest, then return the leg to the start position as you bring the other knee toward your chest. Alternate legs as fast as possible.

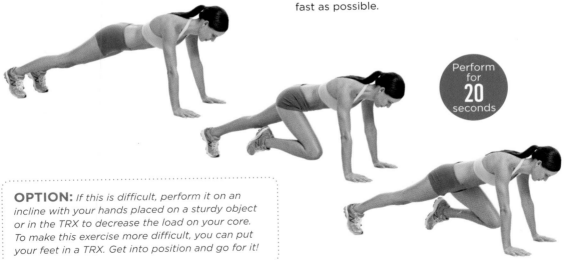

Perform
for
20
seconds

OPTION: *If this is difficult, perform it on an incline with your hands placed on a sturdy object or in the TRX to decrease the load on your core. To make this exercise more difficult, you can put your feet in a TRX. Get into position and go for it!*

PHASE 1: Timed Metabolic Workout

Remember to do the Get Moving RAMP exercises to warm up! Then perform the following exercises one after the other for 30 seconds with 30 seconds of rest between each one. Repeat all five exercises three times and then rest for 3 minutes.

AMAP stands for *as many as possible*! Challenge yourself to push past the number of times you could perform the exercise last time. Feel yourself getting stronger!

Exercise	Sets	Reps	Speed	Rest
CIRCUIT				
1A **Body Weight Squat**	30 secs*	AMAP	Mod	30 secs
1B **Squat Thrust**	30 secs*	AMAP	Mod	30 secs
1C **Alternating Body Weight Reverse Lunge**	30 secs*	AMAP	Mod	30 secs
1D **Prone Hand Touch**	30 secs*	AMAP	Mod	30 secs
1E **Kettlebell or Dumbbell Swing**	30 secs*	AMAP	Mod	30 secs

* Perform all five exercises for 30 seconds each, repeating the circuit three times.

1A Body Weight Speed Squat

Perform as described on page 67. In this workout you're going for speed, but don't get sloppy. Keep your chest up, your knees over your toes, and weight evenly distributed.

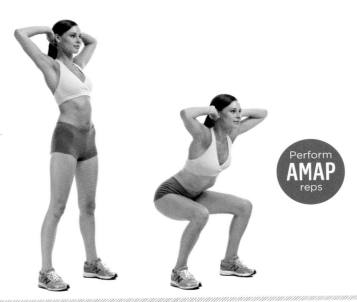

Perform **AMAP** reps

1B Squat Thrust

Combining a squat with a core stabilization movement is the ultimate pairing to really get your heart rate up and burn some calories.

START: Stand with your feet together and your arms at your sides.

MOVEMENT: Bend down and touch the floor with your hands. Put weight on your hands and jump out so your legs are extended into a pushup position, then jump back in so your feet are at your hands again and stand up.

OPTION: *If performing a Squat Thrust on the floor is too difficult, place your hands on a bench or step. The incline will make it easier.*

Perform **AMAP** reps

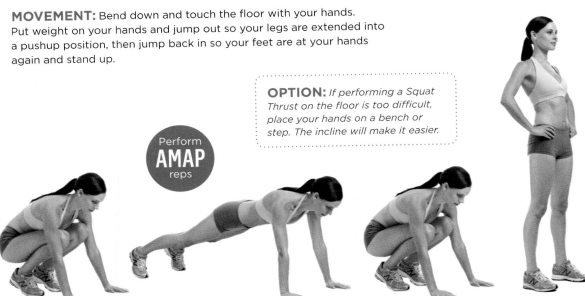

1C Alternating Body Weight Reverse Lunge

You did reverse lunges in the Get Moving RAMP workout—now it's time to push yourself for speed while maintaining your form.

START: Stand up tall with your feet shoulder-width apart, your chest up, shoulders back, head looking straight ahead, and core tight.

MOVEMENT: Keeping your upper body still, shift your weight to one foot and lift the opposite foot behind you, engaging your glute to lift the leg and step back about 2½ feet into a lunge position. Return to the start position and repeat on the opposite leg.

Perform **AMAP** reps

REPEAT on the other side

OPTION: *If the lunge movement is difficult, hold onto the TRX to take some of your body weight off and work on the movement de-loaded.*

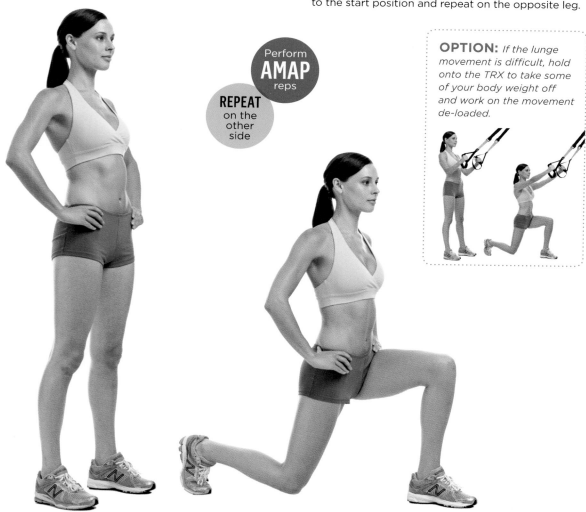

1D Prone Hand Touch

This move has you in the plank position on your hands using your core to stabilize your body. You'll be moving laterally back and forth with your upper body.

START: Get into a pushup position with your body in a straight line.

MOVEMENT: Shift your weight to one hand while keeping your body as stable as possible and quickly touch your free hand to the supporting hand. Place the free hand back in the start position, shift your weight to the other side, and touch your free hand to the supporting hand. Continue back and forth for the entire set.

1E Kettlebell or Dumbbell Swing

If you've never done a swing before, take your time. Start by simply lifting the weight off the floor and setting it back down like a deadlift. Then start to add the swinging motion into the movement.

START: Stand with your feet slightly wider than shoulder-width apart with a kettlebell or dumbbell sitting on the floor just in front of you.

MOVEMENT: Bend down and grab the weight with both hands and hike it between your legs. Stand up by thrusting your hips forward, and swing the weight in front of you to chest height. The key with this exercise is to use your hips and legs rather than your back or arms to get the momentum going to swing the weight. Your weight should be back on your heels, and as you bend your legs, sit back to switch on your glutes. The weight should swing only to chest height. If it's swinging higher than chest height, grab a heavier weight.

Perform **AMAP** reps

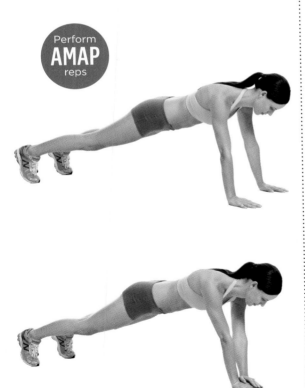

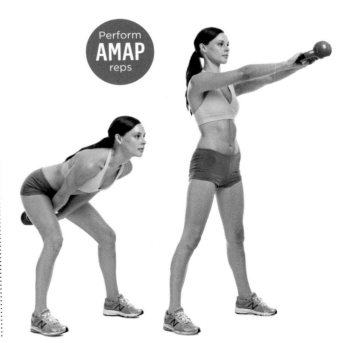

PHASE 1: Countdown Metabolic Workout

Remember to do the Get Moving RAMP exercises to warm up!

Start with 5 reps of each exercise on each side, and then do 4 reps on each side, then 3 reps, then 2, then 1. Jump rope or sprint for 20 seconds at the end of each round. Rest for 2 minutes and repeat for 4 reps, 3 reps, etc.

The next time you perform the countdown workout, add an extra rep (i.e., 6, 5, 4, 3, 2, 1). The third time, add another rep, and so on.

Exercise	*Sets*	*Reps*	*Speed*	*Rest*
CIRCUIT				
1A **Squat Thrust**	5*	5, 4, 3, 2, 1	Mod	30 secs
1B **Body Weight Squat**	5	5, 4, 3, 2, 1	Mod	30 secs
1C **Prone Hand Touch**	5	5, 4, 3, 2, 1	Mod	30 secs
1D **Alternating Kettlebell Clean**	5	5, 4, 3, 2, 1	Mod	30 secs
1E **Alternating Body Weight Reverse Lunge**	5	5, 4, 3, 2, 1	Mod	30 secs
FINISHER				
2 **Jump Rope**	5	20 secs	Mod	2 mins

* Complete all five exercises and jump rope or sprint for one round of declining reps, starting at 5 reps. Repeat whole chart for a total of 5 sets.

PHASE 1 | COUNTDOWN METABOLIC WORKOUT

1A Squat Thrust

See full instructions on page 75.

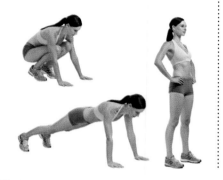

1B Body Weight Speed Squat

See full instructions on page 67.

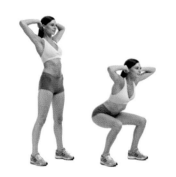

1C Prone Hand Touch

See full instructions on page 77.

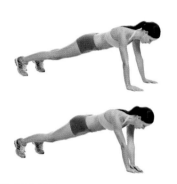

1D Alternating Kettlebell Clean

This exercise involves simply picking the kettlebell up off the floor, then setting it back down and picking it up with the other hand. That's it! The key is to pick it up with your legs and hips; do not round your back.

START: Stand with your feet shoulder-width apart and a kettlebell or dumbbell between your feet.

MOVEMENT: Bend your knees and hips and grab the weight with one hand. In one movement, generating enough power to lift the weight, straighten your legs and stand up, bringing the weight with you all the way up to land on the outside of the forearm. Lower the weight back down by bending your knees and hips to set it back on the floor and then grab it with the opposite hand, repeating the movement on the other side. Alternate back and forth.

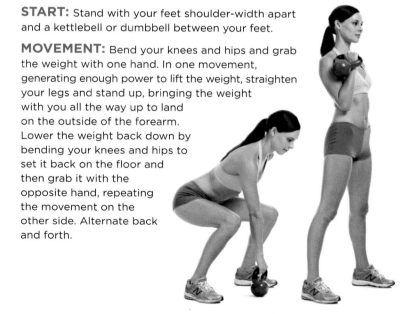

1E Alternating Body Weight Reverse Lunge

See full instructions on page 76.

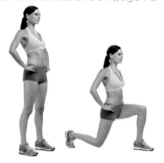

2 Jump Rope or Sprint

If you don't have a jump rope, pretend! Vary your jumps: two feet, one foot at a time, high knees. Stay on the balls of your feet, with knees bent. Or, sprint from one wall to the other.

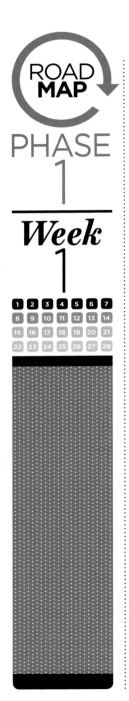

ROAD MAP

PHASE 1

Week 1

This first week focus on just one thing: your mind-set.

Start to catch yourself anytime you think something negative, whether it's "What if I fail and my clothes still don't fit at the end?" or "I'm so far from where I want to be." Know that your body is listening! Break the habit of negative self-talk.

Get your journal out and write your mission statement in the very front. Then write: "I commit . . ." and think through the one action or behavior you can change this week that will have the biggest impact on dropping two sizes. Eliminate sugar? Get more sleep? What one action will make the biggest difference for you this first week? Write it down and then commit to making that change.

Week One Plan of Attack:

After reading Chapter 5, you should have already readied your kitchen and now be ready to take action. Sensitive to dairy? Your grocery list includes milk, yogurt, and cheese as part of the plan. If you find that you are sensitive to dairy, please swap these out for a dairy-free protein option such as almond, soy, or rice products.

Dietary fat does not equal body fat. We have included 2% or full-fat dairy products throughout the plan. You should have some fat with each meal to keep you satiated and because you need some fat. If you choose fat-free milk or yogurt, be sure to add some almonds or other source of good fats to your meal.

Week One Grocery List*

PRODUCE

- **Apples**
- **Bananas**
- **Berries**
- **Pear**
- **Pineapple**
- **Avocado (1)**
- **Bell peppers**
- **Broccoli**
- **Carrots, baby**
- **Celery**
- **Cucumber**
- **Greens, mixed**
- **Mushroom, portobello**
- **Spinach**
- **Sweet potatoes (2)**
- **Tomatoes**
- **Tofu (extra-firm)**

DAIRY & EGGS

- **Cheese, shredded**
- **Eggs**
- **Feta cheese, crumbled**
- **Greek yogurt, 2% (plain)**
- **Milk, 2% (cow, soy, or almond)**

BAKERY

- **Ezekiel bread**

MEAT, DELI & SEAFOOD

- **Chicken breasts, boneless, skinless (1 pound)**
- **Flank steak (5 ounces)**
- **Salmon, wild (6 ounces)**
- **Turkey breast, ground**

GROCERY & PANTRY

- **Ak-mak or RyKrisp crackers**
- **Almonds, raw**
- **Brown rice**
- **Kashi Go Lean cereal**
- **Oatmeal (rolled oats)**
- **Peanut butter, natural**
- **Tuna, canned (in water)**
- **Whey protein powder**

FROZEN

- **Berries**

In addition to the items listed, make sure you have on hand the items listed in "Essential Seasonings & Condiments" on page 43. You'll be using small amounts of these items throughout the next 12 weeks.

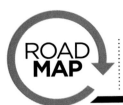

ROAD MAP

Day 1

PHASE 1

Week 1

1	2	3	4	5	6	7
8	9	10	11	12	13	14
15	16	17	18	19	20	21
22	23	24	25	26	27	28

TODAY'S FOCUS ✓

Checkpoint: **Jeans Check**
Pull out the jeans or the outfit you're planning to fit into in 12 weeks and take a picture of how it fits now. Put it somewhere you'll see it every day or exchange "goal" outfits with a friend to hold each other accountable. You will rock your new size soon!

WORKOUT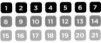

PHASE 1: STRENGTH 1

MENU PLAN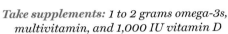

Take supplements: 1 to 2 grams omega-3s, multivitamin, and 1,000 IU vitamin D
Plus 1 serving of Greens+

Breakfast

1 cup cooked oatmeal (made with 1 cup 2% milk)
1 cup fresh berries

Snack

A handful of raw almonds

Lunch

Grilled Chicken Salad: *3 cups mixed greens, 1 cup mixed vegetables (such as cucumber, bell pepper, and tomato), 5 ounces grilled chicken breast, 2 tablespoons Homemade Vinaigrette (page 151)*

Snack

Post-Workout Shake (page 85)

Dinner

6 ounces wild-caught salmon (skin removed), roasted*
2 cups steamed or roasted broccoli
½ cup cooked brown rice

* Brush with Dijon mustard and roast at 400°F for 20-30 minutes until cooked.

Day 2

TODAY'S FOCUS

ACTION: Buddy Up!

Having support is one of the keys to lasting weight loss and improved fitness. You will keep each other accountable and encourage each other to succeed. If you don't have a buddy to join you, decide today that your goal is to inspire someone else throughout your 12-week journey.

You are probably feeling your workout from yesterday. Your inner thighs might be sore from the lateral lunges or your upper body from the overhead press. Let your body recover today.

WORKOUT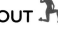

DAY OFF—Active Recovery or complete day of rest

MENU PLAN 🍴

Take supplements: 1 to 2 grams omega-3s, multivitamin, and 1,000 IU vitamin D
Plus 1 serving of Greens+

Breakfast
1 cup 2% Greek yogurt
1 cup cubed pineapple
2 tablespoons chopped raw almonds

Snack
1 apple
2 tablespoons natural peanut butter

Lunch
3 ounces canned (water-packed) tuna mixed with ½ cup chopped celery, 1 tablespoon olive oil mayonnaise, and Dijon mustard to taste
1 pear

Snack
Post-Workout Shake (page 85)

Dinner
4-ounce (cooked) turkey burger in a portobello mushroom
Side Salad: *2 cups mixed greens, 1 cup chopped veggies, and 1 tablespoon Homemade Vinaigrette (page 151)*

Nuts for Nuts!

Unsalted, raw nuts are a good source of many nutrients, including protein, fiber, and healthy fats. In fact, research suggests that eating 1 to 2 ounces daily may help with weight loss. They fill you up without weighing you down! They're perfect for a quick snack that is easy, portable, and doesn't need to be refrigerated. Keep some in your purse, desk, and glove compartment at all times in case you're ever in a pinch. Nuts can be high in fat and calories, but it's the portion we have to watch. A handful—meaning whatever you fit in your cupped hand—is one portion.

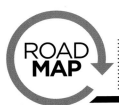

Day 3

PHASE 1

Week 1

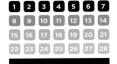

1	2	3	4	5	6	7
8	9	10	11	12	13	14
15	16	17	18	19	20	21
22	23	24	25	26	27	28

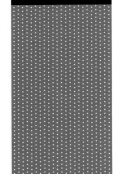

TODAY'S FOCUS ✓

ACTION: Mission Control.
Your mission statement will propel you through this challenge, especially on the days when you start to rationalize giving up or when obstacles arise. Decide today how you will react to them. Will you give up? Or will you stay focused no matter what comes your way? Anticipate problems and be ready!

WORKOUT

PHASE 1: STRENGTH 2

MENU PLAN 🍴

Take supplements: 1 to 2 grams omega-3s, multivitamin, and 1,000 IU vitamin D
Plus 1 serving of Greens+

Breakfast
1 egg + 3 egg whites scrambled with ½ cup fresh vegetables (spinach and bell pepper recommended) and ½ avocado

Snack
1 banana
½ cup 2% Greek yogurt

Lunch
2 slices Ezekiel bread with 2 tablespoons natural peanut butter
A handful of baby carrots

Snack
Post-Workout Shake (page 85)

Dinner
Tofu Stir-Fry*: *2 cups vegetables and 5 ounces diced extra-firm tofu cooked with 2 teaspoons canola oil and low-sodium soy sauce to taste. Serve with ¾ cup cooked brown rice.*

*Make a double batch to have leftovers for lunch on Day 4.

Day 4

TODAY'S FOCUS

Checkpoint: **Water Check**

A simple rule of thumb is to aim for around 8 cups of water per day (or 64 ounces) as a minimum. What will be your strategy to track how much water you drink each day and to make sure you are getting enough?

Use today to recover and regenerate. You're off to a great start! If you are sore from yesterday's workout, take some extra time today to stretch and use a foam roller, The Stick, or a massage ball.

WORKOUT

DAY OFF—Active Recovery or complete day of rest

MENU PLAN

Take supplements: 1 to 2 grams omega-3s, multivitamin, and 1,000 IU vitamin D
Plus 1 serving of Greens+

Breakfast
1 cup Kashi Go Lean cereal
¾ cup fat-free milk
½ banana, sliced

Snack
¼ cup raw almonds

Lunch
1 serving Tofu Stir-Fry (see Day 3)

Snack
Post-Workout Shake (right)

Dinner
5 ounces grilled chicken breast, drizzled with olive oil and a pinch of lemon-pepper seasoning
1 baked sweet potato
Cucumber Salad: 1 cup sliced cucumber topped with thinly sliced red onion, 2 teaspoons extra virgin olive oil, and salt, pepper, and rice vinegar to taste

Post-Workout Shake

1 scoop (20 grams) whey protein powder
1 cup frozen fruit
1 cup fat-free milk, unsweetened almond milk, or soy milk

In a blender, combine the protein powder, fruit, and milk. Blend until smooth. Add water to thin to the desired consistency, if necessary.

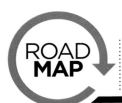

ROAD MAP

PHASE 1

Week 1

1	2	3	4	5	6	7
8	9	10	11	12	13	14
15	16	17	18	19	20	21
22	23	24	25	26	27	28

Day 5

TODAY'S FOCUS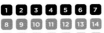

ACTION: Say no, thanks.
Heading into the weekend, remind yourself that every time you stand up to your vices— whether it's a plate of cookies or an extra helping of pasta— you are recommitting to your goals and are one step closer to dropping two sizes. Stand taller, picture yourself wearing your favorite jeans, and say confidently, "No, thank you!"

WORKOUT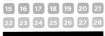

PHASE 1: STRENGTH 1
You should already feel like this workout is easier than it was on Day 1, and you won't be as sore.

MENU PLAN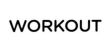

Take supplements: 1 to 2 grams omega-3s, multivitamin, and 1,000 IU vitamin D
Plus 1 serving of Greens+

Breakfast
1 egg + 3 egg whites scrambled with ½ cup fresh vegetables (spinach and bell pepper recommended) and ½ avocado

Snack
1 cup 2% Greek yogurt topped with ½ cup fresh berries

Lunch
3 ounces canned (water-packed) tuna mixed with ½ cup chopped celery, 1 tablespoon olive oil mayonnaise, and Dijon mustard to taste
10 baby carrots
5 ak-mak or RyKrisp crackers

Snack
Post-Workout Shake (page 85)

Dinner
4-ounce (cooked) turkey burger (no bun)
1 baked sweet potato
Side Salad (page 83) and 1 tablespoon Homememade Vinaigrette (page 151)

Day 6

TODAY'S FOCUS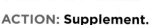

ACTION: Supplement.

You're already a week into the challenge. Congrats! Today's focus is to remember to take a multivitamin and omega-3s as part of your regimen.

A multivitamin guarantees your body has everything it needs to perform optimally, and omega-3s have been shown to benefit your body in a number of ways, including fat oxidation. Even if you are eating lots of fruits, vegetables, and good fats, it is still a good idea to take both supplements.

WORKOUT

TIMED METABOLIC

Today is your first timed metabolic session. Set the clock and get it done!

MENU PLAN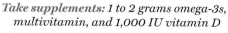

Take supplements: 1 to 2 grams omega-3s, multivitamin, and 1,000 IU vitamin D
Plus 1 serving of Greens+

Breakfast

*1 cup cooked oatmeal
   (made with 1 cup fat-free milk)*
1 cup fresh berries

Snack

1 apple
1 tablespoon natural peanut butter

Lunch

Grilled Chicken Salad (right)

Snack

Post-Workout Shake (page 85)

Dinner

*Omelet made with 3 eggs, ½ cup vegetables,
   and ¼ cup shredded cheese*
1 slice Ezekiel bread

Grilled Chicken Salad

*3 cups
   mixed greens*
*1 cup mixed
   vegetables (such
   as cucumber,
   bell pepper,
   and tomato)*
*5 ounces grilled
   chicken breast*
*2 tablespoons
   Homemade
   Vinaigrette
   (page 151)*

Combine the mixed greens, vegetables, and chicken (or other protein, like steak) and toss with the dressing. Easy, delicious, and healthy!

Day 7

PHASE 1

Week 1

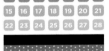

1	2	3	4	5	6	7
8	9	10	11	12	13	14
15	16	17	18	19	20	21
22	23	24	25	26	27	28

TODAY'S FOCUS ✓

ACTION: Get focused.

Plan the next 24 hours and even through the next week. Start to get in the habit of writing out your meals a day ahead in your journal, as well as when you'll do your workouts. Cook meals ahead of time.

WORKOUT

DAY OFF—Active Recovery

Go for a walk or a hike or do something active that you enjoy. Just remember, nothing too taxing. Or you may decide to take the day completely off and relax!

MENU PLAN 🍴

Take supplements: 1 to 2 grams omega-3s, multivitamin, and 1,000 IU vitamin D
Plus 1 serving of Greens+

Breakfast
1 cup Kashi Go Lean cereal
¾ cup 2% milk
½ banana, sliced

Snack
1 apple
A handful of raw almonds

Lunch
2 slices Ezekiel bread with 2 tablespoons natural peanut butter
A handful of baby carrots

Snack
Post-Workout Shake (page 85)

Dinner
Steak Salad: *5 ounces grilled flank steak (thinly sliced), 3 cups mixed greens, ½ cup diced tomato, ¼ cup crumbled feta cheese, 1 tablespoon extra virgin olive oil, and vinegar to taste*

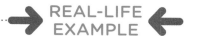
Strong Is the New Beautiful

JOY HILL > dropped three sizes

I had a very specific goal: to get ready to go to the police academy. For the test, I needed to be able to do chinups, pushups, and sprints. I couldn't do any of those things, and even though I was running 3 miles every day, I was not getting any faster and my body's progress had come to a complete halt.

I stopped running and focused on building strength. I overhauled my nutrition habits (I had a mean addiction to Mountain Dew and Flamin' Hot Cheetos) and saw immediate results when I started eating protein and vegetables every few hours and drinking water.

Over 6 months, I transformed my body and was more than ready when it was time to go to the academy. I went from a size 9 to a size 3, gained 7 pounds of muscle and lost 20 pounds of fat, and went from 29 percent body fat to a mean, lean 17 percent.

Being able to do 80 pushups and keep going when everyone else was quitting felt great! I know it was because of the core strength I had built, of which I had ZERO before. I can't believe how many chinups I can do now, and running feels easy when it used to feel hard. I am much faster and feel great!

before   *after*

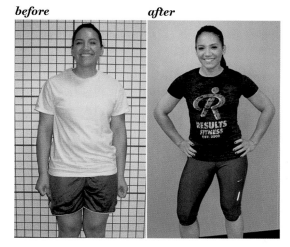

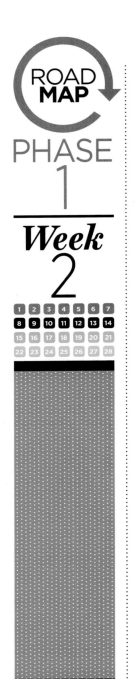

Stay the course as you start Week Two.

Last week you focused on succeeding during this challenge. How did you do? Did you catch yourself throughout the week getting into a negative mind-set or starting to rationalize missing a workout or eating something you weren't planning on? Make your goal this week to get into a routine and plan ahead. Fail to plan, plan to fail.

Each day write out your game plan for the next 24 hours. Your plan can change, but start off with good intentions. Figure out if you need to cook anything ahead of time, run to the store, or lay out your workout clothes so you are ready to go.

Week Two
Plan of Attack:

Decide what you want and why you want it, and understand the changes necessary to reach your goals. Your focus will be on building habits, not breaking habits, and becoming two sizes smaller. You'll become stronger—someone who doesn't make excuses, who knows how to push through obstacles, who doesn't give in.

Your mind has to be conditioned like the rest of your body, and it will strengthen and the challenges will get easier and easier.

Each day, when you open your road map, you'll decide to choose the road that brings you closer to your goal. Ultimately, this path of continuous positive behavior will lead you right back into your favorite clothes (or even a whole new wardrobe)!

Week Two Grocery List

PRODUCE

- Apples
- Bananas
- Pears
- Berries
- Lemons
- Oranges
- Asparagus
- Avocados (2)
- Bell peppers
- Broccoli
- Carrots, baby
- Celery
- Cucumber
- Edamame, shelled (fresh or frozen)
- Garlic
- Greens, mixed
- Spinach
- Sweet potato (1)
- Tomatoes
- Zucchini
- Cilantro
- Hummus

DAIRY & EGGS

- Cheese, shredded
- Cheese, string
- Cottage cheese, low-fat
- Eggs
- Greek yogurt, 2% (plain)
- Milk, 2% (cow, soy, or almond)

BAKERY

- Ezekiel bread
- Ezekiel tortillas

MEAT, DELI & SEAFOOD

- Chicken breasts, boneless, skinless (1¼ pounds)
- Pork tenderloin (¼ pound)
- Salmon, wild-caught (¾ pound)
- Shrimp

GROCERY & PANTRY

- Ak-mak or RyKrisp crackers
- Almond butter
- Almonds, raw
- Black beans (canned, 15 ounces)
- Broth, vegetable or chicken (2 cups)
- Brown rice
- Peanut butter, natural
- Quinoa
- Salsa
- Whey protein powder

FROZEN

- Berries

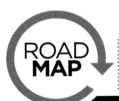

Day 8

PHASE 1

Week 2

1	2	3	4	5	6	7
8	9	10	11	12	13	14
15	16	17	18	19	20	21
22	23	24	25	26	27	28

TODAY'S FOCUS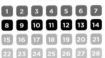

ACTION: Build on your success.
Last week I asked you to pick one thing to change that will get you closer to your goals. What was that one thing? How did you do last week? Were you successful? If you were successful, then keep it up and today choose another change you want to work or improve on. Small changes each week will lead to success. Have a great workout!

WORKOUT

PHASE 1: STRENGTH 2

MENU PLAN 🍴

Take supplements: 1 to 2 grams omega-3s, multivitamin, 1,000 IU vitamin D
Plus 1 serving of Greens+

Breakfast
1 slice Ezekiel bread
2 tablespoons almond butter
1 orange

Snack
¼ cup hummus
10 baby carrots

Lunch
Chicken and Avocado Salad: *3 cups mixed greens topped with 3 ounces grilled chicken, ½ avocado (sliced), ½ cup diced tomato, 1 tablespoon olive oil, and lemon juice to taste*

Snack
Post-Workout Shake (page 85)

Dinner
4 ounces grilled shrimp
2 cups steamed broccoli
¾ cup cooked brown rice

Day 9

TODAY'S FOCUS ✓

ACTION: Be prepared.

It's a good idea to prepare an emergency kit. Always keep a bag of raw unsalted almonds or walnuts and a bottle of water in your purse or car.

WORKOUT

DAY OFF—Active Recovery, optional 20-minute interval session, or repeat metabolic workout

MENU PLAN

Take supplements: 1 to 2 grams omega-3s, multivitamin, and 1,000 IU vitamin D
Plus 1 serving of Greens+

Breakfast

1 cup 2% Greek yogurt
½ cup fresh berries
3 tablespoons chopped raw almonds

Snack

1 apple
2 tablespoons almond butter

Lunch

1 serving Black Bean Soup (See recipe on page 97. You'll use the second serving for lunch on Day 12.)
4 ak-mak or RyKrisp crackers
1 cup fresh fruit

Snack

Post-Workout Shake (page 85)

Dinner

4 ounces roasted or grilled pork tenderloin
2 cups chopped asparagus, roasted with 2 teaspoons olive oil and 1 clove sliced garlic, and sprinkled with salt and pepper

Should You Count Calories?

This challenge is not about counting calories, but losing fat still comes down to the equation:

Calories Eaten < Calories Burned.

If you eliminate most junk food and follow the menus and workouts in this plan, you'll burn more calories than you eat without needing to become obsessive about calorie counting.

There is one caveat: Make sure not to lean too much on foods like nut butters, cheese, and nuts. These are all excellent choices of high-quality protein and good fats, but they can also add up on the wrong side of the calorie equation. Be aware of the foods you choose for snacks and splurges.

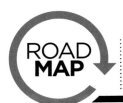

Day 10

PHASE

1

Week

2

1	2	3	4	5	6	7
8	9	10	11	12	13	14
15	16	17	18	19	20	21
22	23	24	25	26	27	28

TODAY'S FOCUS ✅

ACTION: Splurge smart.
Be careful not to waste your splurges on what I call Lazy Cheats. Start to plan out your splurges and use them for something you'll really enjoy, whether it is an experience or something you're really craving. Maybe you like to go to the movies every week and have popcorn or enjoy a cocktail on girls' night out. Don't waste your splurges on "I don't feel like cooking tonight, so I'll have a bowl of cereal for dinner." That's not worth it! Also be careful to count all splurges. For example, "My trail mix only had four M&Ms, so is it still a splurge?" Yes.

WORKOUT 🏋️

PHASE 1: STRENGTH 1

MENU PLAN 🍴

Take supplements: 1 to 2 grams omega-3s, multivitamin, and 1,000 IU vitamin D
Plus 1 serving of Greens+

Breakfast
1 egg + 3 egg whites scrambled with ½ cup fresh vegetables (spinach and bell pepper recommended) and ¼ cup shredded cheese

Snack
1 string cheese
1 pear

Lunch
Asian Chicken Salad: 3 cups mixed greens topped with 3 ounces grilled chicken or shrimp, ½ cup sliced cucumber, ½ cup shelled edamame, ½ cup orange segments, and Sesame Dressing (page 95)

Snack
Post-Workout Shake (page 85)

Dinner
Chicken Burrito: Ezekiel tortilla filled with 3 ounces grilled chicken, ¼ cup diced avocado, ¼ cup cooked brown rice, and salsa
Side Salad (page 83) and 1 tablespoon Homemade Vinaigrette (page 151)

Day 11

TODAY'S FOCUS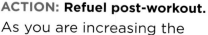

ACTION: Refuel post-workout.
As you are increasing the volume and the intensity of your workouts, it is extremely important that you are taking in something during and/or after your workouts to start the recovery process immediately. Start to get in the habit of bringing with you a blended workout shake that is made up of whey protein and frozen fruit along with milk or water. Plan ahead for your workout tomorrow to prepare a recovery shake to sip during your workout, then finish it when you are done to start the recovery process right away.

WORKOUT

DAY OFF—Active Recovery or complete day of rest

MENU PLAN

Take supplements: 1 to 2 grams omega-3s, multivitamin, and 1,000 IU vitamin D
Plus 1 serving of Greens+

Breakfast
1 cup 2% Greek yogurt
½ cup fresh berries
2 tablespoons chopped raw almonds

Snack
¼ cup hummus
A handful of baby carrots

Lunch
*1 slice Ezekiel bread topped with
    2 tablespoons natural peanut butter*
1 banana

Snack
Post-Workout Shake (page 85)

Dinner
*6 ounces wild-caught salmon
    (skin removed), grilled**
2 cups steamed or roasted broccoli
¾ cup cooked quinoa

**Sprinkle with chili powder or dry rub of
choice and grill for 4 to 5 minutes per side.*

Sesame Dressing

*2 teaspoons
    canola oil*

*1 teaspoon
    sesame oil*

*1 teaspoon honey
    or agave nectar*

*2 teaspoons
    low-sodium
    soy sauce*

Combine the canola oil, sesame oil, honey, and soy sauce and toss with salad.

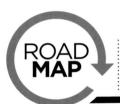

ROAD MAP

PHASE 1

Week 2

1	2	3	4	5	6	7
8	9	10	11	12	13	14
15	16	17	18	19	20	21
22	23	24	25	26	27	28

Day 12

TODAY'S FOCUS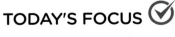

ACTION: Positive produce.
Instead of focusing on what you can't eat this weekend, focus on what you *can*. You can eat all kinds of delicious fruits and vegetables. Take a trip to a farmers' market in your area to pick up local fresh produce.

WORKOUT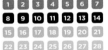

PHASE 1: STRENGTH 2

MENU PLAN

Take supplements: 1 to 2 grams omega-3s, multivitamin, and 1,000 IU vitamin D
Plus 1 serving of Greens+

Breakfast
1 slice Ezekiel bread
2 tablespoons almond butter
1 orange

Snack
1 string cheese
1 pear

Lunch
1 serving Black Bean Soup (see Day 9)
4 ak-mak or RyKrisp crackers
1 cup fresh fruit

Snack
Post-Workout Shake (page 85)

Dinner
5 ounces grilled chicken breast
1 cup cooked zucchini
Side Salad (page 83) and 1 tablespoon Homemade Vinaigrette (page 151)

Day 13

TODAY'S FOCUS

Checkpoint: **Sleep Check**

What are your sleep habits like? Start to make an effort to go to bed at the same time each night and wake up at the same time each morning. Make your room as dark as possible, and stay off the computer and TV right before bed. Sleep is when your body recovers and regenerates.

WORKOUT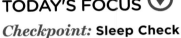

COUNTDOWN METABOLIC

This is your first time doing the Countdown Metabolic Workout—challenge yourself and enjoy!

MENU PLAN

Take supplements: 1 to 2 grams omega-3s, multivitamin, and 1,000 IU vitamin D
Plus 1 serving of Greens+

Breakfast
1 cup chopped fresh fruit
1 cup low-fat cottage cheese
2 tablespoons chopped nuts

Snack
1 apple
1 tablespoon almond butter

Lunch
Chicken and Avocado Salad (page 92)

Snack
Post-Workout Shake (page 85)

Dinner
1 large baked sweet potato topped with 1 cup cooked broccoli and 2 tablespoons plain 2% Greek yogurt
Side Salad (page 83) and 1 tablespoon Homemade Vinaigrette (page 151)

Black Bean Soup

1 tablespoon olive oil
¼ cup chopped carrots
¼ cup chopped celery
Kosher salt and black pepper
2 cups chicken or vegetable broth
1 can (15 ounces) black beans, rinsed and drained, divided
Chopped fresh cilantro

In a saucepan over medium heat, heat the oil. Add the carrots and celery, season with salt and pepper, and cook for 5 minutes, or until lightly browned. Add the broth and half of the beans. Transfer to a blender and blend until smooth. Pour the soup back into the pan and add the reserved black beans and the cilantro.

ROAD MAP

Day 14

PHASE 1

Week 2

1	2	3	4	5	6	7
8	9	10	11	12	13	14
15	16	17	18	19	20	21
22	23	24	25	26	27	28

TODAY'S FOCUS ☑

Checkpoint: **Splurge Check**

Let's keep your momentum going. Take an inventory of your last 2 weeks. Are you following the nutrition recommendations and menus 90 percent of the time? If not, then commit this coming week to improving and planning out your splurges and meals. Cook up your food for the week today so you can hit the ground running tomorrow.

WORKOUT

DAY OFF—**Active Recovery**

Go for a walk or a hike or do something active that you enjoy. Just remember, nothing too taxing. Or take the day completely off and relax!

MENU PLAN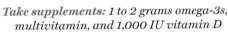

Take supplements: 1 to 2 grams omega-3s, multivitamin, and 1,000 IU vitamin D
Plus 1 serving of Greens+

Breakfast

1 egg + 3 egg whites scrambled with ½ cup fresh vegetables (spinach and bell pepper recommended) and ¼ cup shredded cheese

Snack

¼ cup raw almonds

Lunch

Hummus and Veggie Wrap: *Ezekiel tortilla filled with ¼ cup hummus and 1 cup vegetables*
1 cup fresh fruit

Snack

Post-Workout Shake (page 85)

Dinner

6 ounces wild-caught salmon (skin removed), grilled*
4 cups fresh spinach sautéed with 1 teaspoon olive oil and lemon juice, to taste
¾ cup cooked quinoa

*Sprinkle with chili powder or dry rub of choice and grill for 4 to 5 minutes per side.

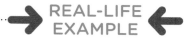
Skinny, But Not Self-Confident

CHRISTINA BLUMER > dropped one size in 8 weeks

I have always thought of myself as an active, healthy young woman. I read package labels when I went grocery shopping, read articles online about the latest nutrition trends, and exercised (not as much as I should have). I would do the standard routine of cardio, then work my upper body one day and lower the next. I was in decent shape but knew there was something missing. I knew I could look better.

Everyone around me was saying things like "You're skinny already! Why are you doing this?" As Rachel says, "It's not about a number on the scale, it's about how you feel in your jeans." That's what this challenge was about for me.

I'm the type of person who needs motivation from multiple sources—to do this challenge on my own would have been impossible. I learned so much about nutrition; about the way the body works and how to set up a series of habits that will stay with me forever. To my friends and family I don't look a whole lot different than I did 12 weeks ago, but I didn't do this for them. I feel great about my body and know I can look even better in time.

In just 3 short months, I dropped a jean size and lost maybe an inch around my waist.

I started this challenge feeling uncomfortable with my body, with low self-esteem, and little hope. Now, my outlook is forever changed. Results don't just get measured on the scale and in the mirror, they go much deeper than that. I cannot wait to see where I can go from here—this is only the beginning.

before   *after*

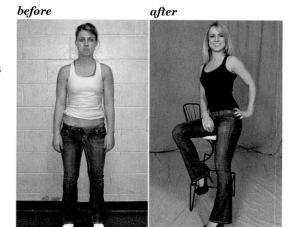

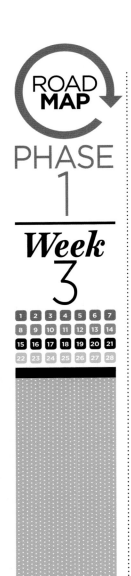

Stay focused in Week Three!

At this point in the program, you may feel yourself slowing down. If you find yourself losing steam, think ahead to next week when you will have your first Jeans Check. Imagine yourself putting on your outfit and the joyful feeling that it's starting to fit!

This week is about reigniting the fire and stepping on the accelerator to get to your destination. Refocus by pulling out your mission statement and revisiting it. Why did you start this challenge again? Why do you want to drop two sizes? How will you feel when you do?

Week Three Plan of Attack:

Remember that this plan is designed to end the cycle of yo-yo dieting! Weight loss programs that don't include strength training may help you lose weight, but a large percentage of that weight is lean muscle tissue. Inevitably, you gain the weight back when the diet ends, and the lost muscle is then replaced with fat.

I consistently see women drop two sizes but only lose, on average, 2 to 4 pounds on the scale. If they had only looked at the scale, they'd be disappointed, but judging by the amazing success stories in this book, I think you'll see why this plan works!

Stick to your strength training and start to feel proud of your strength and ability! Soon enough that feeling will translate to the way you fit into your clothes.

Week Three Grocery List

PRODUCE

- Apples
- Bananas
- Berries
- Oranges
- Pineapple
- Avocado (1)
- Bell peppers
- Broccoli
- Celery
- Cucumber
- Greens, mixed
- Onion, red
- Spinach, baby
- Tomatoes
- Basil
- Tofu (extra-firm)

DAIRY & EGGS

- Cheese, shredded
- Eggs
- Greek yogurt, 2% (plain)
- Milk, 2% (cow, soy, or almond)
- Mozzarella cheese, fresh

BAKERY

- Corn tortillas
- Ezekiel bread
- Ezekiel tortillas

MEAT, DELI & SEAFOOD

- Chicken breasts, boneless, skinless (about 1½ pounds)
- Tilapia (¾ pound)
- Tuna, fresh (¼ pound)
- Turkey breast, ground

GROCERY & PANTRY

- Almonds, raw
- Black beans (canned, 15 ounces)
- Brown rice
- Cranberries, dried, or raisins
- Kashi Go Lean cereal
- Oatmeal (rolled oats)
- Olives, black
- Peanut butter, natural
- Quinoa
- Salsa
- Whey protein powder

FROZEN

- Berries

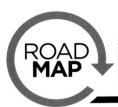

ROAD MAP

Day 15

PHASE 1

Week 3

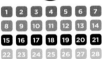

1	2	3	4	5	6	7
8	9	10	11	12	13	14
15	**16**	**17**	**18**	**19**	**20**	**21**
22	23	24	25	26	27	28

TODAY'S FOCUS ✅

Checkpoint: **Brake Check**

Pay attention to what your "brakes" are. Remember that there are three categories: Is it your mind-set? Consistency with your workouts? Or your nutrition? Which of these three is your brake? This week let's release the brakes and take action to accelerate your progress. Really get after your strength workouts. By now you know the exercises, so you can bump up your weights and challenge yourself.

WORKOUT

PHASE 1: STRENGTH 1

MENU PLAN 🍴

Take supplements: 1 to 2 grams omega-3s, multivitamin, and 1,000 IU vitamin D

Plus 1 serving of Greens+

Breakfast

1 cup Kashi Go Lean cereal
¾ cup 2% milk
½ banana, sliced

Snack

1 hard-cooked egg
1 orange

Lunch

Rice Bowl: 1 cup cooked brown rice, ½ cup black beans, 1 cup baby spinach, 3 ounces grilled chicken, and salsa

1 apple

Snack

Post-Workout Shake (page 85)

Dinner

5 ounces cooked tilapia

Caprese Salad: 1 sliced tomato and 2 ounces fresh mozzarella cheese (diced), plus fresh basil leaves, topped with 1 tablespoon extra virgin olive oil and balsamic vinegar to taste

Day 16

TODAY'S FOCUS ✅

Checkpoint: **Veggie Check**
How many servings of veggies a day are you eating? For the first month of the challenge, focus on getting a minimum of three servings of vegetables a day. A serving is about the size of your fist.

WORKOUT

DAY OFF—Active Recovery, optional 20-minute interval session, or repeat metabolic workout from this week.

MENU PLAN

Take supplements: 1 to 2 grams omega-3s, multivitamin, and 1,000 IU vitamin D
Plus 1 serving of Greens+

Breakfast
1 cup cooked oatmeal (made with 1 cup fat-free milk)
½ cup fresh berries

Snack
1 hard-cooked egg
¼ cup raw almonds

Lunch
Chicken Salad Wrap*: *3 ounces cooked chicken breast (shredded or diced) mixed with chopped celery (to taste), sprinkle of Mrs. Dash, 1 tablespoon 2% Greek yogurt, and 1 teaspoon mustard in an Ezekiel tortilla with 1 cup baby spinach*

*Make a double batch of the chicken salad mixture for lunch on Day 18.

1 orange

Snack
Post-Workout Shake (page 85)

Dinner
Tofu Stir-Fry (page 84)

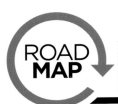

ROAD MAP

Day 17

PHASE 1

Week 3

1	2	3	4	5	6	7
8	9	10	11	12	13	14
15	**16**	**17**	**18**	**19**	**20**	**21**
22	23	24	25	26	27	28

TODAY'S FOCUS

ACTION: Take time for tea.
An easy addition to boost fat burning is to add a cup of green tea a day. Sip your green tea, relax, and know you're another step closer to your goal.

WORKOUT

PHASE 1: STRENGTH 2
Remember today during your workout that the higher your intensity, the higher your metabolism will rev up. Get after it!

MENU PLAN

Take supplements: 1 to 2 grams omega-3s, multivitamin, and 1,000 IU vitamin D
Plus 1 serving of Greens+

Breakfast

Smoothie: *1 banana (frozen if possible), 1 cup 2% Greek yogurt, 1 tablespoon natural peanut butter, and a splash of water (as needed to reach desired thickness)*

Snack

2 tablespoons raw almonds
¼ cup dried cranberries or raisins

Lunch

Grilled Chicken Salad: *3 cups mixed greens, 1 cup mixed vegetables (such as cucumber, bell pepper, and tomato), 5 ounces grilled chicken breast, and 2 tablespoons Homemade Vinaigrette (page 151)*

Snack

Post-Workout Shake (page 85)

Dinner

4 ounces grilled tuna steak
¾ cup cooked quinoa
1 cup steamed broccoli

Day 18

TODAY'S FOCUS ✓

Checkpoint: Attitude Check
Your attitude throughout this challenge is everything. Are you expecting success? Make sure that during your entire workout today, you are focused on how strong and fit you are getting. In your journal, jot down something you wore this week that you felt fabulous in. Remember to keep track of how your clothes fit, not the number on the scale.

WORKOUT

DAY OFF—Active Recovery or complete day of rest.

MENU PLAN

Take supplements: 1 to 2 grams omega-3s, multivitamin, and 1,000 IU vitamin D
Plus 1 serving of Greens+

Breakfast
1 cup Kashi Go Lean cereal
¾ cup fat-free milk
½ banana, sliced

Snack
1 cup 2% Greek yogurt topped with ½ cup fresh fruit

Lunch
1 Chicken Salad Wrap (see Day 16)

Snack
Post-Workout Shake (page 85)

Dinner
Turkey Tacos (right)
Side Salad (page 83) and 1 tablespoon Homemade Vinaigrette (page 151)

Turkey Tacos

5 ounces ground turkey breast
2 teaspoons olive oil
Chili powder (to taste)
2 corn tortillas
1 cup tomato, chopped
¼ cup avocado, diced

Saute the ground turkey in the oil and season with chili powder to taste. Fill corn tortillas with the turkey, then top with the tomato and avocado.

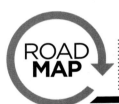

PHASE 1

Week 3

1	2	3	4	5	6	7
8	9	10	11	12	13	14
15	**16**	**17**	**18**	**19**	**20**	**21**
22	23	24	25	26	27	28

Day 19

TODAY'S FOCUS

ACTION: Just say no.

By now the words "No, thank you" should roll right off your tongue! Continue building that habit. It will become easier and easier to tackle those uncomfortable moments. Head into the weekend remembering your three favorite words, "No, thank you."

WORKOUT

PHASE 1: STRENGTH 1

MENU PLAN

Take supplements: 1 to 2 grams omega-3s, multivitamin, and 1,000 IU vitamin D
Plus 1 serving of Greens+

Breakfast
1 cup cooked oatmeal (made with 1 cup fat-free milk)
½ cup fresh berries

Snack
1 hard-cooked egg
1 orange

Lunch
Rice Bowl (page 102)

Snack
Post-Workout Shake (page 85)

Dinner
Tofu Stir-Fry (page 84)

Day 20

TODAY'S FOCUS ✓

Checkpoint: **De-Stress Check**
Are you taking 10 minutes each day to give yourself some downtime? This is an important part of the plan. If you don't give yourself this time to reboot, you'll run yourself down. After your workout today, find something relaxing to do: Take a bath, sit outside, read a book, or meditate.

WORKOUT

TIMED METABOLIC
Push yourself a little harder—can you feel yourself getting stronger?

MENU PLAN

Take supplements: 1 to 2 grams omega-3s, multivitamin, and 1,000 IU vitamin D
Plus 1 serving of Greens+

Breakfast
*1 slice Ezekiel bread topped with
    2 tablespoons natural peanut butter*
1 cup diced pineapple

Snack
*1 cup 2% Greek yogurt topped with
    ½ cup fresh fruit and a drizzle of honey*

Lunch
Grilled Chicken Salad (page 104)

Snack
Post-Workout Shake (page 85)

Dinner
*Pizza: 1 Ezekiel tortilla topped with sliced
    tomato, black olives, thinly sliced
    red onion, and ⅓ cup shredded cheese;
    bake at 350°F until cheese is melted*
*Side Salad (page 83) and 1 tablespoon
    Homemade Vinaigrette (page 151)*

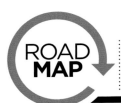

Day 21

PHASE 1

Week 3

1	2	3	4	5	6	7
8	9	10	11	12	13	14
15	**16**	**17**	**18**	**19**	**20**	**21**
22	23	24	25	26	27	28

TODAY'S FOCUS ✓

ACTION: Keep track.
Go back through your journal and add up how many splurges you've used each week. Remember: You're allowed up to three per week. Are you averaging a lot more or a lot less? Make sure to keep your meals balanced and don't overdo it—or deprive yourself.

WORKOUT

DAY OFF—Active Recovery
Go for a walk or a hike or do something active that you enjoy. Just remember, nothing too taxing. Or take the day completely off and relax!

MENU PLAN 🍴

Take supplements: 1 to 2 grams omega-3s, multivitamin, and 1,000 IU vitamin D
Plus 1 serving of Greens+

Breakfast
Smoothie (page 104)

Snack
2 tablespoons raw almonds (or your favorite nut)
¼ cup dried cranberries or raisins

Lunch
Rice Bowl (page 102)

Snack
Post-Workout Shake (page 85)

Dinner
5 ounces cooked tilapia
Caprese Salad (page 102)

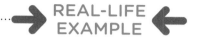
Lasting Changes

ALECIA MENZANO > dropped from size 12 to size 2

I was your typical skinny fat woman. At 5 feet 9 inches tall, I could carry the weight without looking "big," but I wasn't happy. As a former model and professional NFL cheerleader, I wasn't used to being a size 12. I knew I could look and feel better.

I decided to try Drop Two Sizes because I wanted to see if I could fit into a size 8. The challenge kept me focused. I wrote every morsel of food in my journal, I drank all the required water, I worked out (lifted) 3 days a week. I was determined to get into those jeans at the end of the 8 weeks. By the end of the challenge, I was in the jeans, zipped and ready to wear. I weighed in at 150 pounds and 23 percent body fat. I thought that was the end.

A few months later, I put those size 8 jeans on and they felt loose! I couldn't believe it!

I went back to the store and tried on the size 6 and they fit. The last time I was a size 6, I was 18 years old!

It's a year later, and I am now a size 4 (some brands I can wear a 2). I fluctuate between 20 and 22 percent body fat. I have abs! Yes, I can actually see muscles in my stomach. I wear anything I want because I can—I feel great about myself and it shows in everything I do.

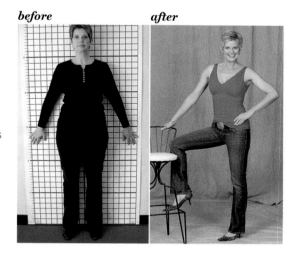

before   *after*

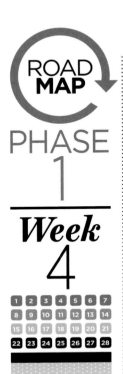

ROAD MAP

PHASE 1

Week 4

1	2	3	4	5	6	7
8	9	10	11	12	13	14
15	16	17	18	19	20	21
22	23	24	25	26	27	28

Week Four is a big moment:

This week you'll try on your jeans! If you've been following the plan, they should fit better already— some of you may even be able to button or zip them up! If you are nervous or don't want to try them on yet, read through some of the stories in this book to find inspiration. Many women started out unsure, just like you!

Now, take a deep breath, and pull them on. I think you'll be pleasantly surprised. Even if you're disappointed in how they feel, you need to know where you stand with your progress. If you don't notice a difference, it is time to step it up.

Week Four Plan of Attack:

Trust the plan in this book. It lays out the exact road map to get you from Point A to Point B. If you're feeling stuck, press your foot on the accelerator and boost your momentum. This week, get as much out of your workouts as you can. Lift a little more weight, do all of the sets, and really push your intensity.

Ask yourself, what one behavior can I work on that will have the biggest impact on my progress to get into my jeans? Use the checkpoints to make sure that you stay on track, and don't take any *wrong turns*. Stay focused on your goals and you'll soon find that you're that much closer to reaching your destination!

Week Four Grocery List

PRODUCE

- Apples
- Bananas
- Lemons
- Melon
- Oranges
- Pears
- Avocado (1)
- Beets
- Bell peppers
- Broccoli
- Carrots, baby
- Celery
- Cucumber
- Eggplant
- Greens, mixed
- Onion, red
- Spinach, baby
- Sweet potato (1)
- Tomatoes
- Zucchini
- Basil

DAIRY & EGGS

- Cottage cheese, low-fat
- Cheese, Laughing Cow
- Cheese, Parmesan
- Cheese, string
- Eggs
- Feta cheese, crumbled
- Greek yogurt, 2% (plain)
- Milk, 2% (cow, soy, or almond)

BAKERY

- Corn tortillas
- Ezekiel bread
- Ezekiel English muffins
- Ezekiel tortillas

MEAT, DELI & SEAFOOD

- Chicken breasts, boneless, skinless (1¼ pounds)
- Flank steak (5 ounces)
- Salmon, wild-caught (6 ounces)
- Turkey breast, ground

GROCERY & PANTRY

- Ak-mak or RyKrisp crackers
- Almonds, raw
- Chickpeas
- Flax seeds, ground
- Pasta, brown rice
- Peanut butter, natural
- Quinoa
- Salsa
- Sunflower seeds
- Tuna, canned (in water)
- Whey protein powder

FROZEN

- Berries

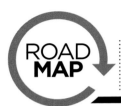

Day 22

PHASE 1

Week 4

1	2	3	4	5	6	7
8	9	10	11	12	13	14
15	16	17	18	19	20	21
22	**23**	**24**	**25**	**26**	**27**	**28**

TODAY'S FOCUS ✓

Checkpoint: **Jeans Check**
Try on your jeans! If you have been sneaking and getting on the scale, then you may not think anything is happening, but I guarantee—if you have been following the program, it is! Write down how you feel about your progress so far in your journal.

WORKOUT

PHASE 1: STRENGTH 2

MENU PLAN

Take supplements: 1 to 2 grams omega-3s, multivitamin, and 1,000 IU vitamin D
Plus 1 serving of Greens+

Breakfast
Breakfast Wrap: *2 scrambled eggs, 1 cup baby spinach, and 2 tablespoons salsa wrapped in an Ezekiel tortilla*

Snack
1 string cheese
1 apple

Lunch
Beet Salad: *3 cups mixed greens, ½ cup chopped cooked beets, ¼ cup crumbled feta cheese, 1 tablespoon extra virgin olive oil, and lemon juice or vinegar to taste*
1 banana

Snack
Post-Workout Shake (page 85)

Dinner
1 cup cooked rice pasta topped with 4 ounces roasted chicken, 1 cup diced tomatoes, ¼ cup Parmesan cheese, and fresh basil

Day 23

TODAY'S FOCUS ✓

Checkpoint: **Attitude Check**

You just tried your jeans on yesterday—they either fit better or they didn't. If you didn't see a difference and have some room to improve, you still have plenty of time. And be careful: If they do fit better, you may catch yourself saying "but . . ."—as in, "They fit better, but I still have a muffin top," or "They're buttoning, but they're still tight on my legs." Stop the negative self-talk! Instead focus on the progress you've made and know that you'll continue to see results going forward!

WORKOUT 🏃

DAY OFF—Active Recovery, optional 20-minute interval session or repeat metabolic workout from this week.

MENU PLAN 🍴

Take supplements: 1 to 2 grams omega-3s, multivitamin, and 1,000 IU vitamin D
Plus 1 serving of Greens+

....

Breakfast

1 slice Ezekiel bread, toasted
2 tablespoons natural peanut butter
1 orange

Snack

2 pieces Laughing Cow cheese
A handful of baby carrots

Lunch

3 ounces canned (water-packed) tuna mixed with ½ cup chopped celery, 1 tablespoon olive oil mayonnaise, and Dijon mustard to taste
5 ak-mak or RyKrisp crackers
1 apple

Snack

Post-Workout Shake (page 85)

Dinner

5 ounces grilled flank steak
1 baked sweet potato
Cucumber Salad: 1 cup sliced cucumber topped with thinly sliced red onion, 2 teaspoons extra virgin olive oil, and salt, pepper, and rice vinegar to taste

The Lazy Cheat

The Lazy Cheat usually starts after a long day of working or running around. You get home just in time for dinner. Tired and famished, you open the fridge, but you really don't feel like cooking, so you decide . . . forget it, let's order pizza!

Occasionally, the Lazy Cheat happens. But it's usually not worth it. You end up using one of your splurges and not really enjoying it. And, unfortunately, once you give in and have a Lazy Cheat, it tends to perpetuate a whole week of them.

The secret to overcoming Lazy Cheats is to have healthy strategies in place. Valerie Waters, celebrity trainer and creator of the Valslide, said, "Strategy trumps willpower." Next time you find yourself tired and hungry, reaching for the take-out menu, turn to the strategy that works to keep you on track.

>> Cont'd on page 115

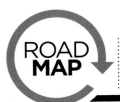

Day 24

PHASE 1

Week 4

1	2	3	4	5	6	7
8	9	10	11	12	13	14
15	16	17	18	19	20	21
22	23	24	25	26	27	28

TODAY'S FOCUS

ACTION: De-emphasize dinner.
Tonight eat a light dinner. The goal is to eat more of your food earlier in the day. If you eat a good breakfast and lunch, you'll be fine with a small dinner. Try it this week. If you find that you are always starving at dinnertime, you probably haven't eaten enough earlier in the day.

WORKOUT

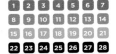

PHASE 1: STRENGTH 1
This is the last time you'll do this routine, so really go for it! Push yourself to get the most out of it before you start a new routine next week.

MENU PLAN

Take supplements: 1 to 2 grams omega-3s, multivitamin, and 1,000 IU vitamin D
Plus 1 serving of Greens+

Breakfast
Breakfast Wrap (page 112)
1 cup diced melon

Snack
1 string cheese
1 apple

Lunch
2 slices Ezekiel bread with 2 tablespoons peanut butter
1 pear

Snack
Post-Workout Shake (page 85)

Dinner
4 ounces cooked chicken breast
2 cups roasted or grilled vegetables (zucchini, eggplant, bell pepper)

Day 25

TODAY'S FOCUS

Checkpoint: **Posture Check**
Stand up straight, pull your shoulders back, engage your stomach muscles, and squeeze your butt. You have been working so hard on building all of these muscles up, so start using them to stand tall every day. Having good posture instantly makes you look like you've lost 10 pounds!

WORKOUT

DAY OFF—Active Recovery or complete day of rest.

MENU PLAN

Take supplements: 1 to 2 grams omega-3s, multivitamin, and 1,000 IU vitamin D
Plus 1 serving of Greens+

Breakfast
1 cup low-fat cottage cheese
1 cup fresh fruit
1 tablespoon ground flax seeds

Snack
2 pieces Laughing Cow cheese
A handful of baby carrots

Lunch
Beet Salad (page 112)
1 banana

Snack
Post-Workout Shake (page 85)

Dinner
*6 ounces wild-caught salmon
   (skin removed), roasted**
2 cups steamed or roasted broccoli
¾ cup cooked quinoa

*Brush with mustard and roast at 400°F for 20 minutes.

The Lazy Cheat

>> Cont'd from page 113

Keep menus on hand of go-to restaurants where you know you can get a healthy meal. I have a whole stack of menus in my car. If I've had a busy day with no plan for dinner, I'll call ahead and place an order, then pick it up on my way home.

Replace Lazy Cheats with Easy Meals that you fall back on at these times. One of my Easy Meals is a chicken breast with a can of lentil soup. I grill up the chicken breast, heat up the soup, and pour it over the chicken breast—done!

It's also okay just to have a healthy shake for dinner. Blend up a scoop of protein powder and some fruit or peanut butter, and enjoy.

Plan out your week ahead of time, including your splurges. Your week should include 10 percent of meals where you can indulge—so don't waste them!

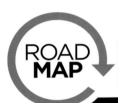

ROAD MAP

Day 26

PHASE 1

Week 4

1	2	3	4	5	6	7
8	9	10	11	12	13	14
15	16	17	18	19	20	21
22	23	24	25	26	27	28

TODAY'S FOCUS

ACTION: Snack smart.

What are you leaning on too much? Nuts? Nut butter? Cheese? Are you finding yourself grabbing one of these more often than you should be? If so, then it's time to cut back and find a different option. One of my clients said, "No more scooping." She was referring to the multiple spoonfuls of peanut butter she ate each day. Look through the menus and get new ideas instead of scooping or grabbing a hunk of cheese. A handful of raw almonds is an excellent snack.

WORKOUT

PHASE 1: STRENGTH 2

This is your last time on this program. Really push yourself!

MENU PLAN

Take supplements: 1 to 2 grams omega-3s, multivitamin, and 1,000 IU vitamin D
Plus 1 serving of Greens+

Breakfast
1 slice Ezekiel bread, toasted
1 tablespoon natural peanut butter
1 orange

Snack
A handful of raw almonds

Lunch
3 ounces canned (water-packed) tuna mixed with ½ cup chopped celery, 1 tablespoon olive oil mayonnaise, and Dijon mustard to taste
A handful of baby carrots
5 ak-mak or RyKrisp crackers

Snack
Post-Workout Shake (page 85)

Dinner
1 cup cooked rice pasta topped with 4 ounces roasted chicken, 1 cup diced tomatoes, ¼ cup Parmesan cheese, and fresh basil

Day 27

TODAY'S FOCUS

ACTION: Put supplements front and center.

Have you been taking your multivitamin and omega-3 supplements every day? This is an easy action step that is also easy to forget. Keep the bottles handy in your kitchen or bathroom where you'll see them every day. Make it a priority.

WORKOUT

COUNTDOWN METABOLIC

MENU PLAN

Take supplements: 1 to 2 grams omega-3s, multivitamin, and 1,000 IU vitamin D
Plus 1 serving of Greens+

Breakfast

1 cup Greek yogurt topped with 1 cup fresh fruit and 1 tablespoon sunflower seeds

Snack

2 pieces Laughing Cow cheese
A handful of baby carrots

Lunch

2 slices Ezekiel bread with 2 tablespoons peanut butter
1 pear

Snack

Post-Workout Shake (page 85)

Dinner

4-ounce cooked turkey burger in an Ezekiel English muffin
Side Salad (page 83) and 1 tablespoon Homemade Vinaigrette (page 151)

Chicken Fajitas

2 teaspoons
    canola oil
6 ounces boneless,
    skinless chicken
    breast, cut into
    strips
½ red onion, sliced
1 bell pepper, sliced
Kosher salt
Ground black
    pepper
2 corn tortillas
Salsa

In a large skillet over medium-high heat, heat the oil. Add the chicken, onion, and bell pepper; season with salt and black pepper and cook for 10 to 12 minutes, or until the chicken is cooked through. Serve the chicken mixture wrapped in tortillas, with salsa. Makes 1 serving.

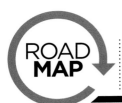

Day 28

PHASE 1

Week 4

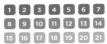

1	2	3	4	5	6	7
8	9	10	11	12	13	14
15	16	17	18	19	20	21
22	**23**	**24**	**25**	**26**	**27**	**28**

TODAY'S FOCUS ✅

ACTION: Treat yourself!.
You've completed 1 month on this plan. Congratulations! Use the great feeling today to motivate you for Month Two. Read through your new workout for the coming week, shop and prepare for your meals, and get ready to attack the week. Take some time today to do something to reward yourself—perhaps get a pedicure or buy a new workout outfit. You have done fantastic so far and deserve a treat. Indulge a little today.

WORKOUT 🏃

DAY OFF—Active Recovery or take a complete day of rest. Enjoy!

MENU PLAN 🍴

Take supplements: 1 to 2 grams omega-3s, multivitamin, and 1,000 IU vitamin D
Plus 1 serving of Greens+

Breakfast
1 cup low-fat cottage cheese
1 cup fresh fruit
1 tablespoon sunflower seeds

Snack
A handful of raw almonds

Lunch
Avocado and Chickpea Salad: *3 cups mixed greens, ½ cup chickpeas, ½ cup sliced cucumber, ½ cup diced avocado, ½ cup chopped bell pepper, 1 tablespoon extra virgin olive oil, and lemon juice or vinegar to taste*

Snack
Post-Workout Shake (page 85)

Dinner
Chicken Fajitas (page 117)

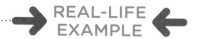
Stay the Course

LYNNEA CLARK > dropped two sizes in 12 weeks

When I started Drop Two Sizes, I had 20 pounds of pregnancy weight to lose, and at 46 years of age, my metabolism isn't what it used to be. The first week of the challenge wasn't difficult because it was new and I was determined to get off to a brilliant start. But by Week Two, I was a little discouraged about facing 11 more weeks of the plan. I slipped up when I ate five homemade cookies and some larger meal portions at the end of the week.

By Week Three, I started coming to the gym every day and found out that motivated me more. I can't always stand up to hunger, but working out every morning was something I felt I had more control over.

Drop Two Sizes explains how, in our culture, we tend to want things now. I needed to throw out that mind-set.

Not being allowed to step on the scale helped me to focus on hitting my stride and not get caught up with the invariable fluctuations of weight readings that can so often be confusing and discouraging. I embraced the change, and the results followed!

before   *after*

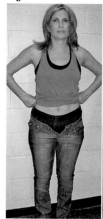
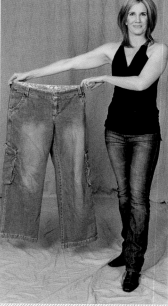

PHASE TWO

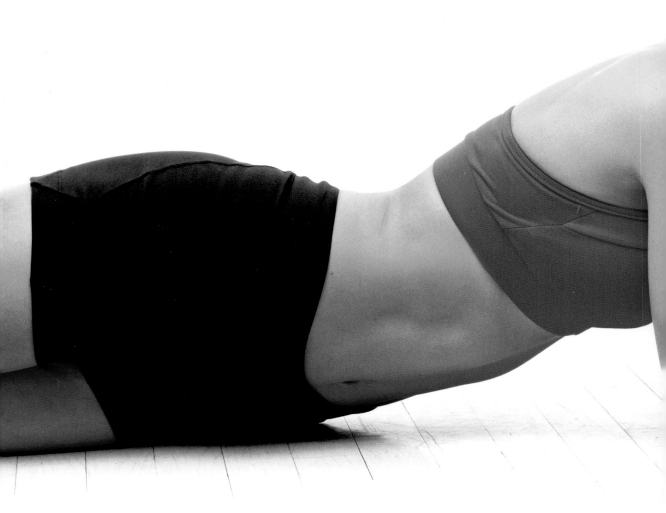

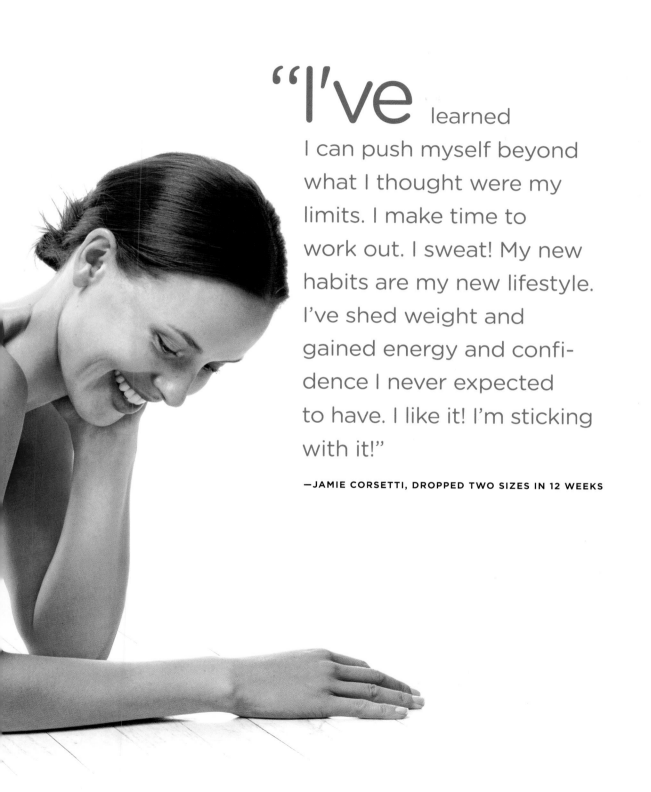

"**I've** learned I can push myself beyond what I thought were my limits. I make time to work out. I sweat! My new habits are my new lifestyle. I've shed weight and gained energy and confidence I never expected to have. I like it! I'm sticking with it!"

—JAMIE CORSETTI, DROPPED TWO SIZES IN 12 WEEKS

Congratulations on completing the first month of this plan! You have started to build great habits and should notice a significant difference in the wa y your clothes fit now. As you move into the next phase of the training, remember all the things you've learned and continue to apply them on a day-by-day basis.

PHASE 2:
Road Maps

Read through the following weekly road maps before you get started, and then go through them again each week as you follow the plan. Commit to following the next 30 days of this plan as closely as possible. Get yourself hooked on feeling fit, rather than focusing on trying to reach a number on the scale by the end of the second month.

PHASE 2:
Menu Plan

You've made it through the first 30 days of this plan; built strong, healthy habits; and set up successful strategies to continue on this path over the next 8 weeks and beyond. But that's not to say things are any easier now! At about this point, I usually hear complaints from my clients that they are getting bored with eating

the same foods. This book offers fantastic menus specifically designed to keep you interested and help you avoid getting stuck in a rut. If you feel yourself getting bored and eating the same thing every day, try a new recipe or add a new vegetable into your menu during this phase.

Remember: You may not be able to stick to the menus exactly, and that's okay. Do the best you can, but feel confident in your ability to swap meals or repeat those you know work with your schedule and preferences.

GOALS OF PHASE 2:

→ *Continue with the momentum you've built in Phase One.*

→ *Stay focused now that the starting line is long behind you and the finish line still seems off in the distance.*

→ *Bump up your vegetables to 6 to 8 servings a day.*

PHASE 2: **Workouts**

The following is your plan for the next 4 weeks. It's laid out here to make sure you can plan ahead and make time for all the workouts, to achieve the best possible results. Do not add anything, change anything, or skip anything. All you need to do is commit to taking it one day at a time!

	Monday	Tuesday	Wednesday	Thursday	Friday	Saturday	Sunday
Week 5	**Day** 29 STRENGTH WORKOUT 1	**Day** 30 DAY OFF: Active Recovery or optional 20-minute interval session	**Day** 31 STRENGTH WORKOUT 2	**Day** 32 DAY OFF: Active Recovery	**Day** 33 STRENGTH WORKOUT 1	**Day** 34 TIMED METABOLIC	**Day** 35 DAY OFF: Active Recovery
Week 6	**Day** 36 STRENGTH WORKOUT 2	**Day** 37 DAY OFF: Active Recovery or optional 20-minute interval session	**Day** 38 STRENGTH WORKOUT 1	**Day** 39 DAY OFF: Active Recovery	**Day** 40 STRENGTH WORKOUT 2	**Day** 41 COMPLEX METABOLIC	**Day** 42 DAY OFF: Active Recovery
Week 7	**Day** 43 STRENGTH WORKOUT 1	**Day** 44 DAY OFF: Active Recovery or optional 20-minute interval session	**Day** 45 STRENGTH WORKOUT 2	**Day** 46 DAY OFF: Active Recovery	**Day** 47 STRENGTH WORKOUT 1	**Day** 48 TIMED METABOLIC	**Day** 49 DAY OFF: Active Recovery
Week 8	**Day** 50 STRENGTH WORKOUT 2	**Day** 51 DAY OFF: Active Recovery or optional 20-minute interval session	**Day** 52 STRENGTH WORKOUT 1	**Day** 53 DAY OFF: Active Recovery	**Day** 54 STRENGTH WORKOUT 2	**Day** 55 COUNT-DOWN METABOLIC	**Day** 56 DAY OFF: Active Recovery

PHASE 2: RAMP

Perform one set of each of the following warmup exercises before you start each workout.

1 **Foam Roller/Self-Myofascial Release Full Body**

2 **Hip Flexor/TFL Stretch**
(Hold 30 seconds on each side)

3 **Marching Hip Bridge** (8 reps, holding for 1 second at the top of each rep)

4 **Quadruped Hydrant** (8 reps on each side)

5 **Bent-Over Reach to Sky**
(8 reps on each side)

6 **Squat to Stand 1** (8 reps)

7 **Scapular Pushup** (8 reps)

8 **Toe-Raised Ankle Mobility** (8 reps)

9 **Forward/Backward Jump** (10 reps)

10 **Alternating Single Leg Romanian Deadlift** (8 reps on each side)

11 **Lateral Jump** (8 reps)

12 **Cross-Behind Lunge** (8 reps on each side)

13 **Dynamic Lunge with Overhead Reach**
(8 reps on each side)

14 **Lateral Shuffle** (8 reps on each side)

RAMP 1: Foam Roller/ Self-Myofascial Release

Hopefully you purchased a foam roller for your home (or a lacrosse ball, which can be used as a massage ball). These tools work great to massage your muscle without having to fork over big bucks for a professional masseuse.

As you go through the RAMP stretches and movements on the following pages, notice where you feel tight—you can use the foam roller or ball to massage that area. Eventually you can work through your entire body. In addition, you can roll out your tensor fascia latae (TFL) and iliotibial (IT) band by lying on your side and rolling the outside of your leg from your hip to your knee. This tends to be a pretty sore spot, but you'll be glad you did it!

Your muscles will probably be tender the first time you roll them out, so don't push through any pain if it becomes excruciating. If it is so painful that you're tensing up, the exercise won't work as designed. Each time you use the foam roller it should feel less uncomfortable. Ideally, you'll want to use the foam roller a few minutes each day.

Use it regularly to avoid injury and feel great after your workouts! Focus on rolling out 3 to 5 areas that feel tight.

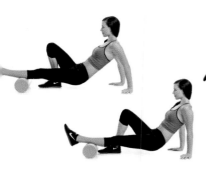

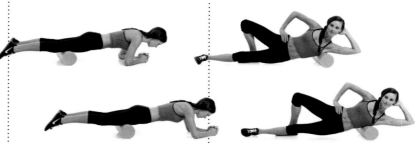

Calves

POSITION: Place your left calf on the roller and support yourself, putting as much weight on the calf as you can. Turn your left leg in and roll so you are massaging the inside of your left calf. Then turn your toe straight up and roll and finish with your toe turned out. Repeat on the opposite leg.

Quads

POSITION: Roll right over so the roller is on the tops of the fronts of your legs and lean to one side. Roll up and down and then switch to the other side.

Lats

POSITION: Lie on the roller so that it is under your armpit, and roll from your armpit to your hip along your lat with your bottom arm extended or bent behind your head.

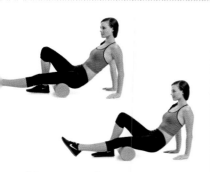

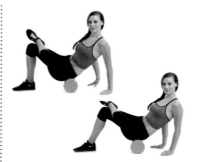

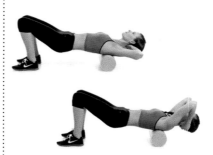

Hamstrings

POSITION: With your leg straight out and your hands behind you with your weight back on your arms, roll from the top of your leg where your hamstring goes into your hip right down to your knee. Put your weight on one leg and roll up and down, and then massage the other leg.

Hips

POSITION: Sit on the foam roller, cross your left leg over your right, and lean toward your left hip, putting your weight on your left hand. Roll on your glute and stop if you feel a spot that feels like a knot. Switch sides.

Thoracic Mobilization

POSITION: With the foam roller across your upper back, place your hands behind your head to support your neck. With your elbows up and out, roll slowly up and down your upper back as you extend and relax back onto the roller.

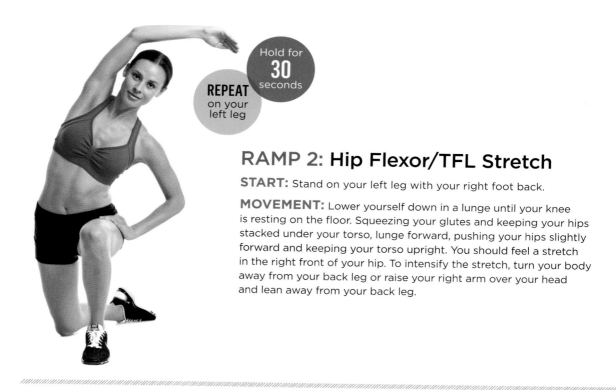

Hold for 30 seconds

REPEAT on your left leg

RAMP 2: Hip Flexor/TFL Stretch

START: Stand on your left leg with your right foot back.

MOVEMENT: Lower yourself down in a lunge until your knee is resting on the floor. Squeezing your glutes and keeping your hips stacked under your torso, lunge forward, pushing your hips slightly forward and keeping your torso upright. You should feel a stretch in the right front of your hip. To intensify the stretch, turn your body away from your back leg or raise your right arm over your head and lean away from your back leg.

RAMP 3: Marching Hip Bridge

START: Lie on your back with your knees bent and your feet flat on the floor. Lift your hips off the floor to form a straight line from your shoulders to your knees. Your arms should be on the floor with your palms facing up.

MOVEMENT: Maintaining that straight line, lift your right leg, then return it to the starting position and lift your left leg, and continue alternating. As you lift one leg, your opposite hip will want to drop, but keep your gluteal (butt) muscles contracted the entire time to hold your hips square. It's as if you're marching while keeping your hips extended. This is to wake up your glutes.

Perform 8 reps

Hold 1 second

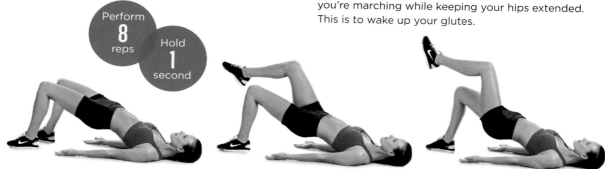

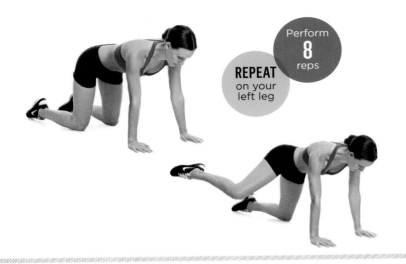

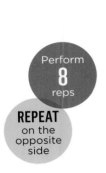

Perform **8** reps

REPEAT on your left leg

RAMP 4: Quadruped Hydrant

This is a progression from the Side Lying Clam Shell in Phase One.

START: Get down on the floor on your hands and knees.

MOVEMENT: Keeping your elbows straight, raise your right leg out to the side. Move only at your hip, not your lower back. Repeat to finish your reps. Continue with the opposite leg.

RAMP 5: Bent-Over Reach to Sky

START: Stand with your feet shoulder-width apart. Bend over at your waist with your back in a neutral position and your knees slightly bent. Your arms should hang straight down in front of you with your palms facing each other.

MOVEMENT: Keeping your arms straight, lift one arm out toward the ceiling as you rotate your torso around to look at the ceiling. Your hand will be pointing straight up to the ceiling with your palm facing out, while the opposite hand remains pointing straight down to the floor. Return to the start position.

Perform **8** reps

REPEAT on the opposite side

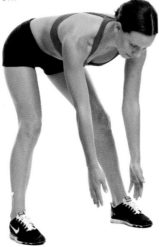

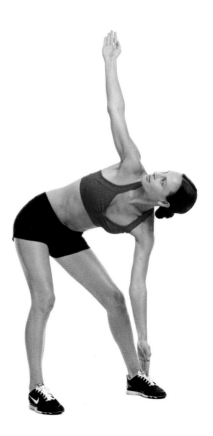

RAMP 6:
Squat to Stand 1

START: Stand with your feet slightly wider than shoulder-width apart.

MOVEMENT: Bend over at your waist to touch the floor between your feet, keeping your legs straight and stretching out your hamstrings. Keeping your hands on the floor, drop your hips down into a squat position. From here, stand up to return to the start position and repeat.

Perform
8
reps

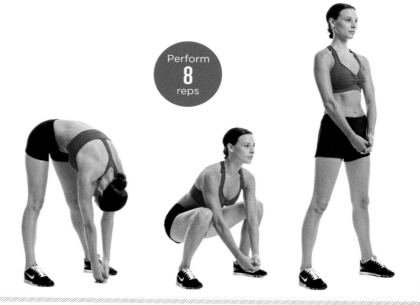

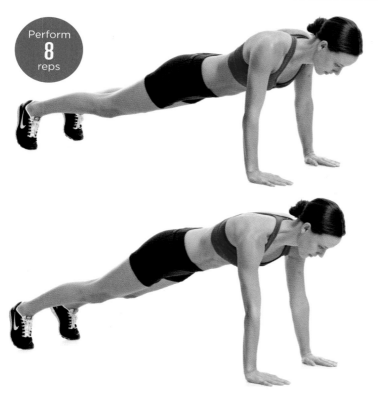

Perform
8
reps

RAMP 7:
Scapular Pushup

START: Get in a pushup position with your body in a straight line, hips down and core engaged, and arms straight.

MOVEMENT: Keeping your arms straight and your spine long, push your body up by protracting your shoulder blades (taking them farther away from your spine). Then retract your shoulder blades by pulling them toward your spine and feel your body lower again without bending your arms. Repeat, making sure not to let the tension creep up into your shoulders and neck.

RAMP 8:
Toe-Raised Ankle Mobility

START: Fold up your mat or a towel or use a weight plate to raise your toes up about an inch high with your heels on the floor.

MOVEMENT: Keeping your heels on the floor, slightly bend your knees over your fourth and fifth toes to stretch your ankles and calves.

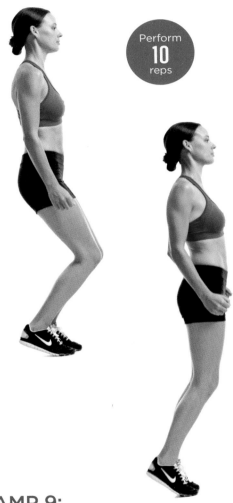

Perform
10
reps

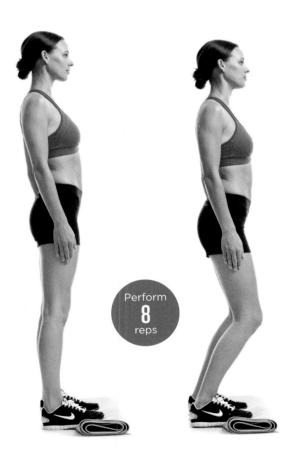

Perform
8
reps

RAMP 9:
Forward/Backward Jump

START: Stand with your feet together. Imagine a line running horizontally in front of you.

MOVEMENT: Jump over the line, landing on both feet. Then jump backward over it to the start. Keep the jumps small and pretend the floor is hot. This exercise will really wake up your nervous system!

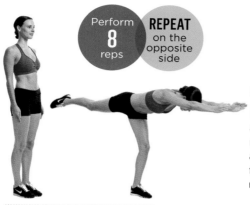

Perform 8 reps   **REPEAT on the opposite side**

RAMP 10: Alternating Single Leg Romanian Deadlift

START: Stand with your feet shoulder-width apart.

MOVEMENT: Shift your weight to balance on one leg with a slight bend in the knee of the standing leg. Bend at your hip, reaching your free leg back as you reach your arms forward and feel the movement of keeping your hips square to the floor as you bend from the hip. Return to the start position and repeat on the opposite side, alternating back and forth.

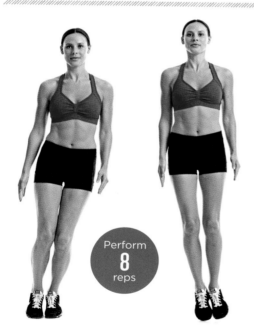

Perform 8 reps

RAMP 11: Lateral Jump

START: Stand with your feet together. Imagine there is a line to your right.

MOVEMENT: With both feet, jump up and over the line and land on both feet. Pretend the floor is hot so you will land and immediately jump right back over to the other side of the line. Keep your knees bent the entire time, exploding back and forth. Wake up your nervous system!

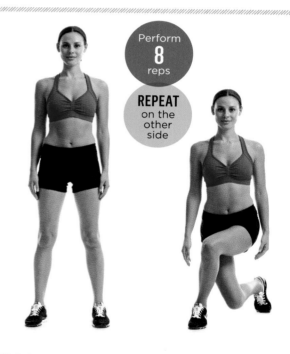

Perform 8 reps   **REPEAT on the other side**

RAMP 12: Cross-Behind Lunge

START: Stand with your feet shoulder-width apart and your arms at your sides.

MOVEMENT: Cross your left foot over your right and step about 2 feet to the right of your right foot. Bend both knees, in a movement very similar to a curtsy. Keep your hips facing forward. You should feel a stretch across your left hip as you lunge. Return to the start position and repeat on the other side.

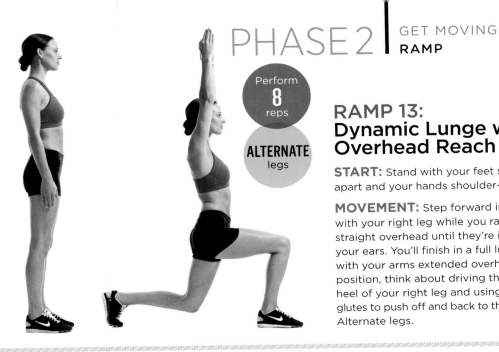

Perform 8 reps

ALTERNATE legs

RAMP 13:
Dynamic Lunge with Overhead Reach

START: Stand with your feet shoulder-width apart and your hands shoulder-width apart.

MOVEMENT: Step forward into a lunge with your right leg while you raise your arms straight overhead until they're in line with your ears. You'll finish in a full lunge position with your arms extended overhead. From this position, think about driving through the heel of your right leg and using your leg and glutes to push off and back to the start position. Alternate legs.

RAMP 14:
Lateral Shuffle

START: Stand with your feet facing forward, wider than shoulder-width apart, and knees bent.

MOVEMENT: Shuffle one foot to the other, moving laterally while keeping your knees bent, staying low with feet facing straight forward. Always keep at least a foot between your feet while moving. Don't let your feet come together. Continue in one direction for 3 to 5 shuffles and then switch directions.

Perform 8 reps

SWITCH directions

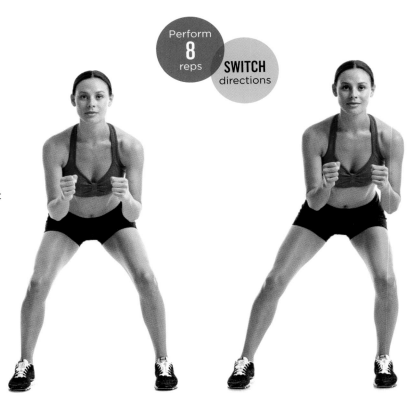

PHASE 2: Strength
Workout 1

Remember to do the Get Moving RAMP exercises to warm up! Then perform the following exercises as described in the chart.

Exercise	Sets	Reps	Speed	Rest
CORE				
1 TRX Fallout	1-2	8	Mod	45 secs
POWER				
2 Push Press	2-3	8	Fast	1 min
STRENGTH				
3A Offset Dumbbell Front Squat	2-4	8-10, alternate sides each set	Mod	1 min
3B Bench Plank Single Arm Dumbbell Row	2-4	8-10 each side	Slow	None
3C Marching Hip Bridge	2-4	8-10 each side	Mod	None
4A Single Leg Romanian Deadlift	2-4	8-10 each side	Slow	1 min
4B Pushup	2-4	8-10	Slow	None
4C Toe-Raised Ankle Mobility	2-4	8-10	Mod	None
FINISHER				
5 Lunge Step Over to Isometric Lunge	2-4	20 secs work	20 secs hold	20 secs rest

1 TRX Fallout

This exercise may not look like much, but you'll feel it in your core tomorrow.

START: With your hands holding a TRX, reach your arms straight out and drop your hips so that your hips, back, shoulders, and head are in a straight line and your arms are extended overhead next to your ears. This is the "end" position, but it works best to start here so you know your range of motion.

MOVEMENT: From that end position, maintaining a neutral spine and keeping your body as stable as you can, bring your arms down to the top of a pushup position, keeping them straight. Return to the start position and then repeat.

OPTION: *If you don't have access to a TRX, you can do this exercise with your knees on a ball. Another option, if you don't have a TRX or a ball, is to go back to the plank exercise from Phase One and lift alternating arms in the plank position.*

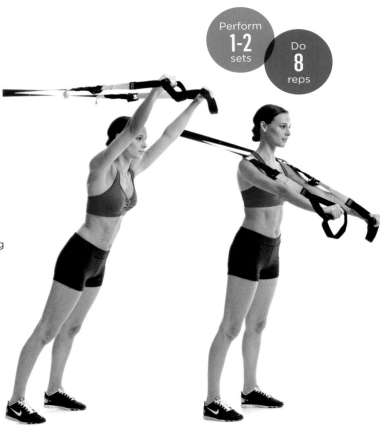

Perform **1-2** sets Do **8** reps

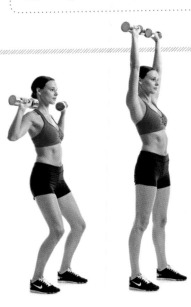

2 Push Press

This exercise looks like an upper-body exercise, but you are actually lifting a weight that you need to use your lower body to explode up and lift. This is all about generating power from your entire body. And as the weight lands overhead, your core must switch on to support it. So your upper body, lower body, and core will all benefit! Plus, you'll feel your heart rate pumping from the explosive movement.

Perform **2-3** sets Do **8** reps

START: Stand holding two dumbbells on your shoulders.

MOVEMENT: Using the momentum from your legs, start with a small bend and then explode up and push the dumbbells overhead. Return to the start position and repeat. This is an explosive movement and should be done with a weight that you could not simply press up with your arms alone.

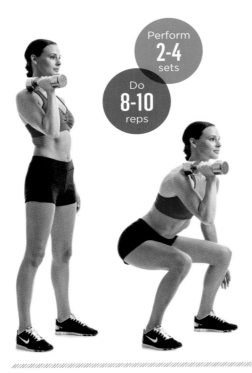

Perform
2-4
sets

Do
8-10
reps

3A Offset Dumbbell Goblet Squat

Carrying something on one side of your body is a part of life. We very rarely lift and carry something with two hands. Usually we lift a bag of groceries and carry it on our hip as we open a door or carry a kid on one side or lug around our purses that weigh about 20 pounds. It is important to train movements we will do in our real lives. This is one of those movements.

START: Hold a dumbbell in one hand. Stand with your feet slightly wider than shoulder-width apart, toes pointing slightly out, and core engaged with good posture. Bend your elbow so the dumbbell is resting at shoulder height with your wrist straight to support the weight.

MOVEMENT: Bend your hips and knees to lower into a squat, keeping your body centered by fighting the offset load. Your weight should stay even on both legs, and your heels should stay down. Try to get your hips below parallel. Then return to the start position. Perform all on one side, and switch sides on your next set.

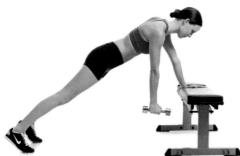

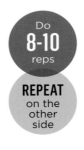

Do
8-10
reps

REPEAT
on the
other
side

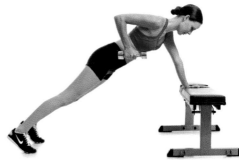

3B Bench Plank Single Arm Dumbbell Row

Here's that "plank" position again. With all these planks your core is going to be so strong. Did someone say "flat tummy"?

START: With one hand on a bench or step and the other hand holding a dumbbell, walk your feet out so your body is in a straight line, creating a plank position with your shoulders, hips, and ankles in line and the dumbbell hanging straight down.

MOVEMENT: Keeping your body stable and your shoulders down, row the dumbbell by pulling your elbow up alongside your body. Think about using your upper back to pull the weight up by pulling your shoulder blade back and down. Lower the dumbbell back to the start position and repeat. When you have finished the repetitions, switch sides.

3C Marching Hip Bridge

Perform as described on page 126.

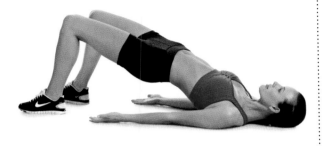

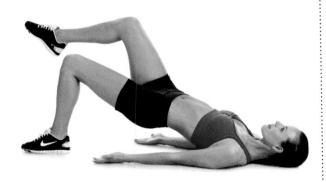

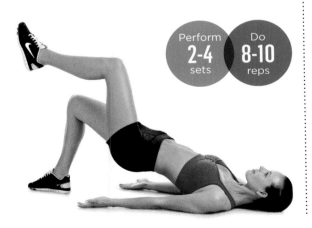

Perform **2-4** sets

Do **8-10** reps

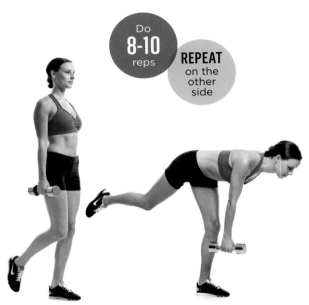

Do **8-10** reps

REPEAT on the other side

4A Single Leg Romanian Deadlift

This is one of my favorite exercises for working your butt and the back of your legs. You are also getting the added benefit of strengthening your core and the shoulder of the arm holding the weight.

START: Practice the movement first without holding a weight by balancing on your left leg with a slight bend in the knee. Bend at your hip, reaching your right leg back and grazing the floor as a kickstand, reaching your right hand toward the floor while keeping your back neutral. Feel the movement of keeping your hips square to the ground as you push back into your hips. Once you are able to do this, hold a dumbbell or kettlebell in your right hand.

MOVEMENT: Keeping your hips square and your back neutral (do not round your back), balance on one leg and slowly lower the dumbbell toward the floor by bending at your hip. Return to the start position. Repeat. Switch legs.

4B **Pushup**

Perform as described on page 71.

Perform **2-4** sets Do **8-10** reps

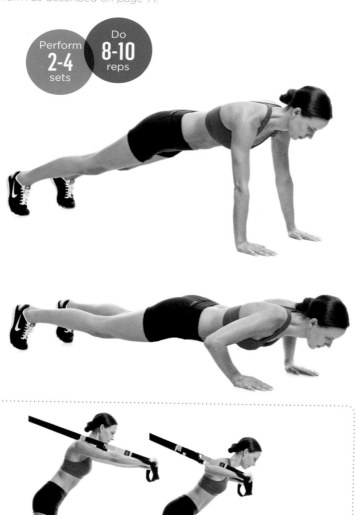

OPTION:
Perform the pushup on an incline, either on a TRX or on a bench or step.

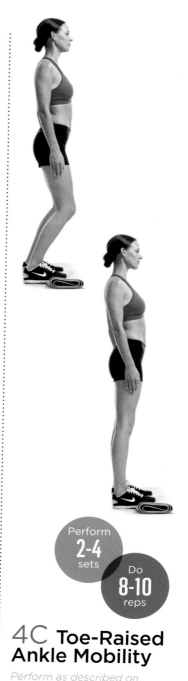

Perform **2-4** sets Do **8-10** reps

4C **Toe-Raised Ankle Mobility**

Perform as described on page 129.

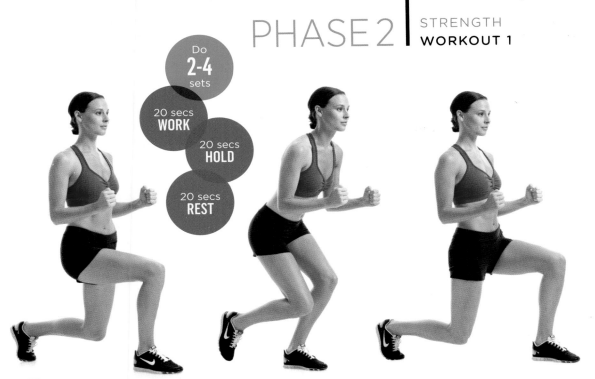

Do
2-4
sets

20 secs
WORK

20 secs
HOLD

20 secs
REST

5 Lunge Step Over to Isometric Lunge

This one will burn your legs. Commit to maintaining good posture, keeping your body as upright as you can, and keeping the working leg under tension without taking a break. Mind over matter with this one. Enjoy!

START: Get into a lunge position with your body upright.

MOVEMENT: Stay low with your legs under tension and bring your back leg through to the front to lunge with the opposite stance. Bring it back through to the start. Your standing leg is your working leg and should stay under tension the entire time without standing up to rest. Next, hold the bottom of the lunge position for 20 seconds. Then rest and repeat on the opposite leg.

OPTION: *If the standard exercise is too difficult, hold on to a TRX to take some of your body weight off to make it easier by de-loading the exercise.*

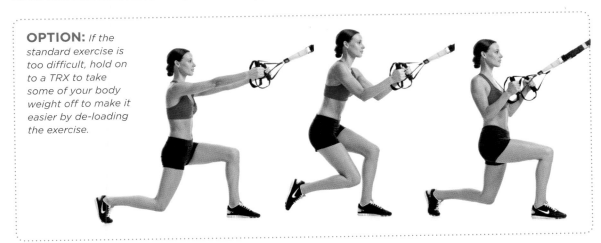

PHASE 2: Strength
Workout 2

Remember to do the
Get Moving RAMP exercises
to warm up!

Exercise	Sets	Reps	Speed	Rest
CORE				
1 Half-Kneeling Halo	1-2	5 ea direction	Mod	45 secs
COMBINATION				
2 Alternating Clean to Squat Thrust	2-3	4 ea side	Fast	1 min
STRENGTH				
3A Rear-Foot Elevated Split Squat	2-4	8-10 ea side	Mod	1 min
3B Single Arm Standing Overhead Press	2-4	8-10 ea side	Slow	None
3C Hip Flexor/ TFL Stretch	2-4	30 secs each	Hold	None
4A Suitcase Deadlift	2-4	8-10 ea side	Slow	1 min
4B TRX Inverted Row	2-4	8-10	Slow	None
4C Bent-Over Reach to Sky	2-4	8 ea side	Slow	None
FINISHER				
5 Body Weight Squat with Isometric Squat Hold	2-4	20 secs move	20 secs hold	20 secs

1 Half-Kneeling Halo

This is a really fun core exercise!

START: Get into a half-kneeling position, which you learned in your Get Moving RAMP Workout: Balance on one knee with the other foot in line with your back knee in a "Will you marry me?" pose. Your posture should be upright, with your core engaged and your hips stacked under your shoulders. Hold a dumbbell or a kettlebell in front of your chest with both hands.

MOVEMENT: Continuing to hold the weight with both hands, bring it around to one side, then behind your head and back to where you started to form a full circle. As you perform the movement, keep your body still with your core engaged and your glutes switched on. Alternate sides, performing 5 reps in each direction, and then switch legs.

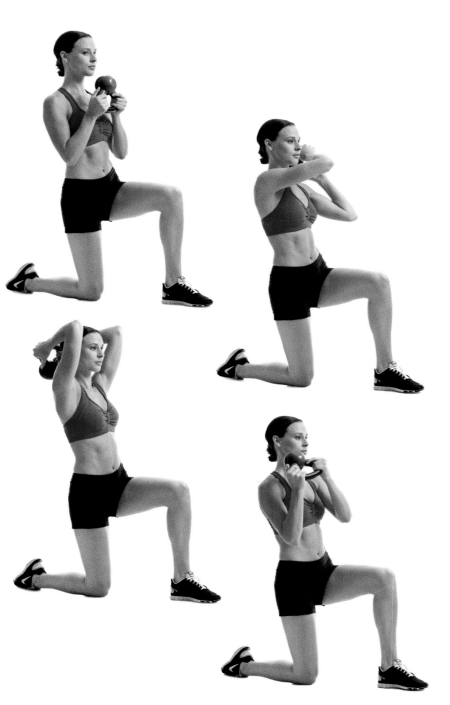

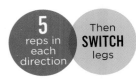

5 reps in each direction

Then **SWITCH** legs

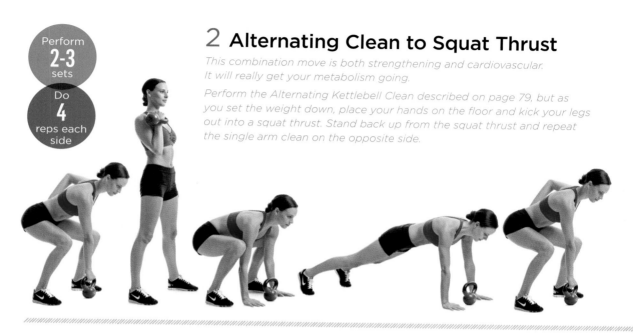

Perform
2-3
sets

Do
4
reps each
side

2 Alternating Clean to Squat Thrust

*This combination move is both strengthening and cardiovascular.
It will really get your metabolism going.*

*Perform the Alternating Kettlebell Clean described on page 79, but as
you set the weight down, place your hands on the floor and kick your legs
out into a squat thrust. Stand back up from the squat thrust and repeat
the single arm clean on the opposite side.*

3A Rear-Foot Elevated Split Squat

*This is one of the most hated but most effective exercises in
my gym. I usually tell my clients to "hate me now, but love me
later when you're wearing jeans that are two sizes smaller!"
This exercise works the entire leg while giving the other leg an
excellent stretch. As the exercise gets easier hold dumbbells
to make it more challenging.*

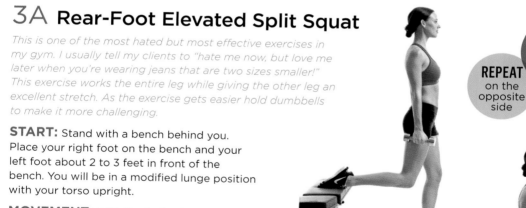

Perform
8-10
reps

REPEAT
on the
opposite
side

START: Stand with a bench behind you.
Place your right foot on the bench and your
left foot about 2 to 3 feet in front of the
bench. You will be in a modified lunge position
with your torso upright.

MOVEMENT: With the bulk of your body
weight on your left leg, bend your left knee
until your thigh is below parallel and your right
knee is grazing the floor. Keep your weight
on your left leg. Don't sit back and put weight
on your right leg—that's cheating. Pause in
this position and then return to a fully upright
position. Repeat for the desired number of
reps and then continue on the opposite side.

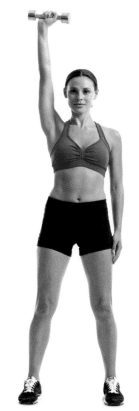

3B Single Arm Standing Overhead Press

Build some shoulders while you shrink your hips. Any time you press a weight overhead, your core is working. With the offset load on this exercise, it will be working overtime.

START: Stand with your feet shoulder-width apart, knees slightly bent, and hips right underneath your shoulders. Hold a dumbbell in one hand resting at shoulder height.

MOVEMENT: Press the dumbbell overhead, keeping your butt and abs tight to keep your body stable. Resist the urge to lean to one side. Extend your arm all the way up overhead and then lower under control back to the start position. Repeat for the desired number of reps on the same arm. Then switch sides.

Perform **8-10** reps

REPEAT on the opposite side

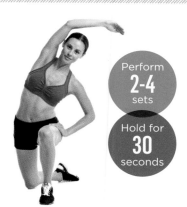

Perform **2-4** sets

Hold for **30** seconds

3C Hip Flexor/ TFL Stretch

Perform as described on page 126.

4A Suitcase Deadlift

START: Stand with your feet shoulder-width apart with a dumbbell or kettlebell in one hand at your side.

MOVEMENT: Bend down, keeping your shoulders even. Lower down as far as you can while maintaining a neutral back. Stand up straight as though picking up a suitcase. Repeat for the desired number of reps.

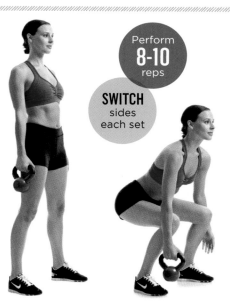

Perform **8-10** reps

SWITCH sides each set

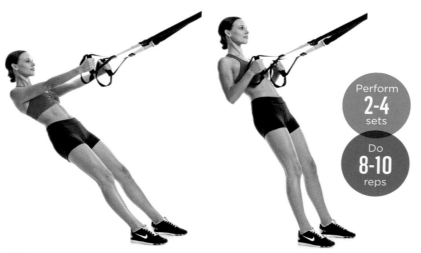

Perform
2-4
sets

Do
8-10
reps

OPTION: *If you don't have a TRX, you can perform an inverted row with a bar securely placed on a squat rack. Lying on the floor, hold on to the bar and pull yourself up. If that's not an option, you'll have to substitute a different rowing motion, such as a Bent-Over Dumbbell Row.*

4B TRX Inverted Row

Although this exercise focuses primarily on working the muscles of the back in the rowing movement, it is a great total body exercise. It is one of those most bang for your buck exercises I mentioned earlier. You'll feel your legs, butt, core, and upper body working hard.

START: Hold the handles of your TRX and walk underneath so you are hanging your body weight from the TRX with your feet straight out and your body in a straight line. Lift your hips so your body is completely flat. Your position should look like an upside-down pushup. If this position is too difficult, walk up higher to have less of an incline.

MOVEMENT: Perform a rowing motion, using your upper back to pull your body up by pulling your elbows back and squeezing your shoulder blades back and together. Keep your body completely straight throughout the entire motion. To progress the exercise, position your feet farther under the TRX until you are almost on the floor. To continue progressing, put your feet up on a step or bench.

4C Bent-Over Reach to Sky

Perform as described on page 127.

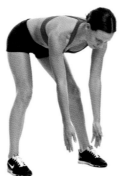
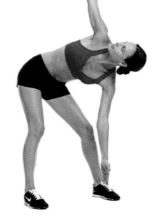
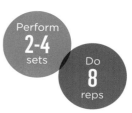

Perform
2-4
sets

Do
8
reps

5 Body Weight Squat with Isometric Squat Hold

Perform the Body Weight Squats according to the description on page 79 for the required time period and then hold the bottom position, which is the Isometric Squat Hold.

Perform
2-4
sets

SQUAT
20 secs

HOLD
20 secs

REST
20 secs

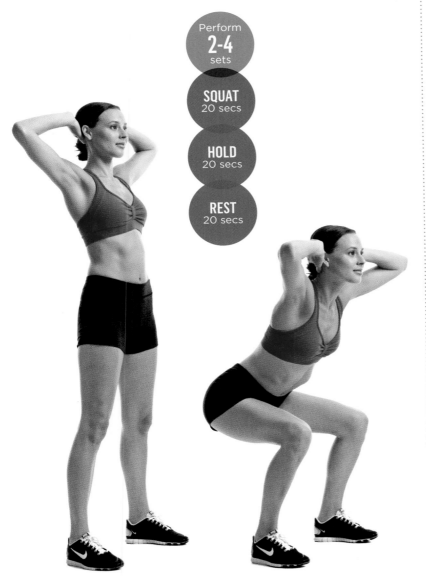

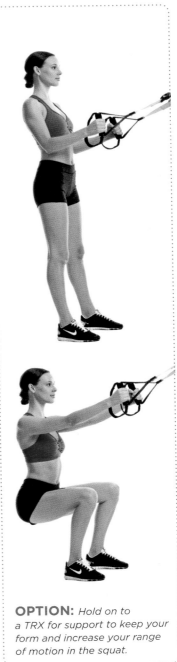

OPTION: *Hold on to a TRX for support to keep your form and increase your range of motion in the squat.*

PHASE 2: Timed
Metabolic Workout

First do the Get Moving RAMP exercises. Then perform the following exercises one after the other for 40 seconds of work with 20 seconds of rest between each one.

Repeat these five exercises for 40 seconds on, 20 seconds rest, 3 times and then rest for 2 to 3 minutes.

Exercise	Sets	Reps	Speed	Rest
CIRCUIT				
1A Dumbbell Swing	3 secs	AMAP	Mod	20 secs
1B Alternating Lateral Lunge	3 secs	AMAP	Mod	20 secs
1C Alternating Bent-Over Dumbbell Row	3 secs	AMAP	Mod	20 secs
1D Reverse Lunge with Overhead Reach	3 secs	AMAP	Mod	20 secs
1E Alternating T-Stabilization	3 secs	AMAP	Mod	20 secs
REST				
Active Recovery		Rest for 2-3 min		

1A Dumbbell Swing

See full instructions on page 77.

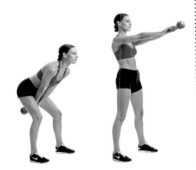

1B Alternating Lateral Lunge

START: Stand with your feet shoulder-width apart.

MOVEMENT: Step with your right leg into a lateral lunge, keeping your back in a neutral position with your chest up. Drive off that outside leg to return to the start position and then immediately step out into a lateral lunge with your left leg. Repeat, alternating back and forth for the entire set.

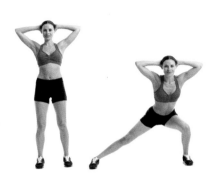

1C Alternating Bent-Over Dumbbell Row

START: Hold a dumbbell in each hand and bend over at your hips with your back in a neutral position and your knees slightly bent.

MOVEMENT: Keeping your body still, row one dumbbell up and then the other, alternating back and forth.

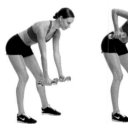 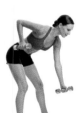 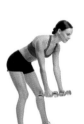 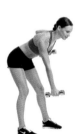

1D Reverse Lunge with Overhead Reach

See full instructions on page 61.

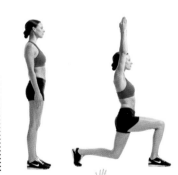

1E Alternating T-Stabilization

See full instructions on page 63.

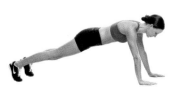

PHASE 2: Complex
Metabolic Workout

First do the Get Moving RAMP exercises. Then perform 8 of each of the following exercises one after the other, moving as fast as possible. Rest for 90 seconds and then repeat. Perform four rounds.

Exercise	Sets	Reps	Speed	Rest
CIRCUIT				
1A Dumbbell Alternating Reverse Lunge	4	8	Fast	None
1B Romanian Deadlift	4	8	Fast	None
1C High Pull	4	8	Fast	None
1D Front Squat to Push Press	4	8	Fast	None
REST				
Active Recovery	Rest for 90 secs			

1A Dumbbell Alternating Reverse Lunge

START: Stand tall with your feet shoulder-width apart and a dumbbell in each hand.

MOVEMENT: Step back into a reverse lunge and then drive through your front leg to return to the start position. Repeat on the opposite leg. Continue alternating back and forth.

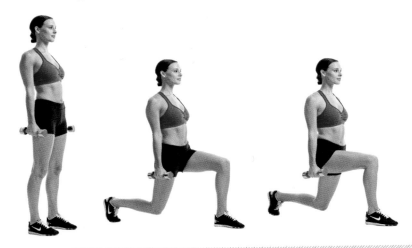

1B
Romanian Deadlift

See full instructions on page 70.

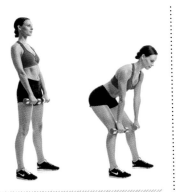

1C
High Pull

See full instructions on page 64.

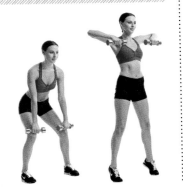

1D Front Squat to Push Press

Holding a dumbbell in each hand at shoulder height, perform a Goblet Squat according to the description on page 133. As you come out of the bottom squat, generate enough power to explode the weight you are holding overhead into a push press. Lower the weight carefully to the shoulders and repeat.

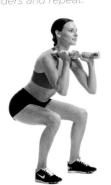

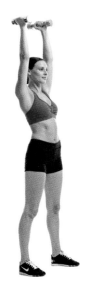

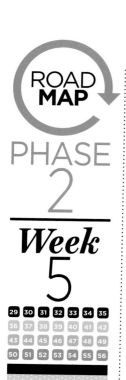

Welcome to Week Five!

Now that you've made it through the first 30 days of the plan, you've started to change old habits and build new behaviors—hopefully they're starting to feel like a part of your daily routine. But at this point in the plan I often start hearing complaints from my clients that sound like, "I'm getting bored eating the same foods."

If you're feeling stale or growing tired of any aspect of the plan, use this week to shake things up. Since this is a road map for the rest of your life, you need to keep things interesting so you'll stay motivated. You'll have all new workouts this week, so get ready to attack those with a fresh start. And enjoy experimenting in the kitchen!

Week Five
Plan of Attack:

Challenge yourself to try new meals and commit to getting creative. Read through the Menu Plans and recipes and pick out something for each day that you haven't eaten before. Do whatever it takes to make meals that keep you interested and excited.

Check out the essential seasonings and condiments list on page 43 and try them out on various recipes. Take notes in your journal so you can remember what you liked or any surprisingly good combinations! Even if you don't consider yourself a chef, you can enjoy preparing meals that help you stick to your goals. Food is fuel and will help you feel fabulous!

Week Five Grocery List

PRODUCE

- Bananas
- Grapefruit
- Lemons
- Melon
- Oranges
- Pineapple
- Avocado (1)
- Broccoli
- Carrots
- Celery
- Cucumber
- Edamame, shelled (fresh or frozen)
- Greens, mixed
- Onion, red
- Spinach, baby
- Sweet potato (1 small)
- Tomatoes
- Tomatoes, cherry
- Cilantro (optional)

DAIRY & EGGS

- Cheese, Laughing Cow light
- Cheese, shredded
- Eggs
- Greek yogurt, 2% (plain)
- Milk, 2% (cow, soy, or almond)
- Orange or grapefruit juice, 100%

BAKERY

- Corn tortillas
- Ezekiel bread
- Ezekiel tortillas

MEAT, DELI & SEAFOOD

- Chicken breasts, boneless, skinless (1¼ pounds)
- Pork tenderloin
- Salmon, wild-caught (⅓ pound)
- Shrimp
- Turkey breast, ground

GROCERY & PANTRY

- Ak-mak or RyKrisp crackers
- Almond butter
- Almonds, raw
- Black beans, canned (15 ounces)
- Broth, vegetable or chicken
- Brown rice
- Kashi Go Lean cereal
- Olives, black
- Quinoa
- Salmon, canned
- Salsa
- Whey protein powder

FROZEN

- Berries

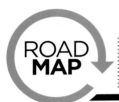

Day 29

PHASE 2

Week 5

29	30	31	32	33	34	35
36	37	38	39	40	41	42
43	44	45	46	47	48	49
50	51	52	53	54	55	56

TODAY'S FOCUS ✔

Checkpoint: Splurge Check
Go through your journal and tally up your splurges. Are you averaging three a week? More? If you overdid it during the first month, you can make up for that now by using fewer than three splurges this week. For example, if you had 16 splurges last month, reduce your weekly splurges to two each week this month.

WORKOUT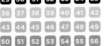

PHASE 2: STRENGTH 1
You have all new strength workouts today, so focus on getting to know the new exercises. Perform only two sets of each exercise today.

MENU PLAN 🍴

Take supplements: 1 to 2 grams omega-3s, multivitamin, and 1,000 IU vitamin D
Plus 1 serving of Greens+

Breakfast
Smoothie: *1 cup 2% Greek yogurt, ½ grapefruit*

Snack
*2 tablespoons almond butter
10 celery sticks*

Lunch
*1 serving Black Bean Soup (page 97). You'll use the second serving for lunch on Day 33.
5 ak-mak or RyKrisp crackers*

Snack
Post-Workout Shake (page 85)

Dinner
Chicken Pizza*: *1 Ezekiel tortilla topped with sliced tomato, black olives, thinly sliced red onion, ⅓ cup shredded cheese, and 3 ounces cooked chicken breast*

*Bake at 400°F until cheese is melted.
Side Salad (page 83) and 1 tablespoon Homemade Vinaigrette (Day 30)

Day 30

TODAY'S FOCUS ✅

ACTION: Rock your new habits!
You have made it to the 30th day of the challenge! You rock! It takes anywhere from 21 to 30 days to build a new habit. At this point, you should start to feel like healthy nutrition and exercise have become an important part of your lifestyle.

WORKOUT

DAY OFF: Active Recovery
optional 20-minute interval workout, or repeat the metabolic workout from this week

MENU PLAN 🍴

Take supplements: 1 to 2 grams omega-3s, multivitamin, and 1,000 IU vitamin D
Plus 1 serving of Greens+

Breakfast
2 eggs (any style)
1 slice Ezekiel bread, toasted
1 cup diced melon or other fresh fruit

Snack
A handful of raw almonds
Sliced cucumber (unlimited)

Lunch
3 ounces canned salmon mixed with ½ cup chopped celery, 1 tablespoon olive oil mayonnaise, and Dijon mustard to taste
3 cups mixed greens + ½ cup cherry tomatoes

Snack
Post-Workout Shake (page 85)

Dinner
Chicken Burrito (page 94)

Homemade Vinaigrette

Making your own salad dressing is a great, healthy alternative to eating fat- and calorie-laden store-bought dressings. All you need are two simple ingredients that, when combined, offer just as much flavor and zing!

¾ cup extra virgin olive oil
¼ cup balsamic vinegar

Mix the olive oil and vinegar well, and drizzle over greens.

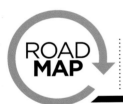

ROAD MAP

PHASE

2

Week

5

29	30	31	32	33	34	35
36	37	38	39	40	41	42
43	44	45	46	47	48	49
50	51	52	53	54	55	56

Day 31

TODAY'S FOCUS

ACTION: Try something new.
Pick out one new recipe and make it today! Cooking and preparing meals is an ongoing journey, and you'll want to continue exploring new foods to keep things interesting and fun. If you're stuck in a rut of eating broccoli as your vegetable every night, try something completely different like bok choy, or mash up some steamed cauliflower.

WORKOUT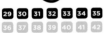

PHASE 2: STRENGTH 2

MENU PLAN

Take supplements: 1 to 2 grams omega-3s, multivitamin, and 1,000 IU vitamin D
Plus 1 serving of Greens+

Breakfast
1 cup 2% Greek yogurt
½ cup fresh fruit
3 tablespoons chopped raw almonds

Snack
2 pieces Laughing Cow light cheese
5 ak-mak or RyKrisp crackers

Lunch
Asian Chicken Salad (page 94)
    and Sesame Dressing (page 95)

Snack
Post-Workout Shake (page 85)

Dinner
4 ounces grilled shrimp
2 cups steamed broccoli
¾ cup cooked brown rice

Day 32

TODAY'S FOCUS

Checkpoint: **Veggie Check**
Have you been eating a minimum of three servings a day? As of this week, bump your vegetables up to a minimum of four servings a day.

WORKOUT

DAY OFF: Active Recovery
or complete day of rest.

MENU PLAN

Take supplements: 1 to 2 grams omega-3s, multivitamin, and 1,000 IU vitamin D
Plus 1 serving of Greens+

Breakfast
1 cup Kashi Go Lean cereal
¾ cup fat-free milk
½ banana, sliced

Snack
2 tablespoons almond butter
10 celery sticks

Lunch
Rice Bowl (page 102)

Snack
Post-Workout Shake (page 85)

Dinner
Turkey Tacos (page 105)

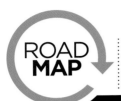

Day 33

PHASE

2

Week

5

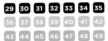

29	30	31	32	33	34	35
36	37	38	39	40	41	42
43	44	45	46	47	48	49
50	51	52	53	54	55	56

TODAY'S FOCUS ✅

ACTION: Plan ahead.

What is your plan for the weekend? Figure out your strategies today to be prepared. The weekend tends to be the hardest time for most people because it's a break from the normal routine. Take time to think through potential obstacles and have solutions in mind so you can tackle any situation with ease.

WORKOUT

PHASE 2: STRENGTH 1

MENU PLAN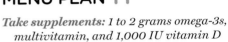

Take supplements: 1 to 2 grams omega-3s, multivitamin, and 1,000 IU vitamin D
Plus 1 serving of Greens+

Breakfast
Smoothie: *1 cup 2% Greek yogurt, ½ grapefruit*

Snack
A handful of raw almonds

Lunch
1 serving Black Bean Soup (page 97)
5 ak-mak or RyKrisp crackers
1 cup fresh fruit

Snack
Post-Workout Shake (page 85)

Dinner
4 ounces roasted or grilled pork tenderloin
1 small baked sweet potato
2 cups steamed spinach topped with 1 teaspoon olive oil and lemon juice, to taste

Day 34

TODAY'S FOCUS

ACTION: Reward yourself.

You've been pushing your body like an athlete and working out hard. Are you taking time to recover, too? This includes stretching, foam rolling or other self-massage, and rest. Think about booking yourself a massage at a spa as a reward.

WORKOUT

PHASE 2: TIMED METABOLIC

MENU PLAN

Take supplements: 1 to 2 grams omega-3s, multivitamin, and 1,000 IU vitamin D
Plus 1 serving of Greens+

Breakfast
2 eggs (any style)
1 slice Ezekiel bread, toasted
1 cup fresh fruit

Snack
2 pieces Laughing Cow light cheese
5 ak-mak or RyKrisp crackers

Lunch
3 ounces canned salmon mixed with ¼ cup chopped celery, 1 tablespoon olive oil mayonnaise, and Dijon mustard to taste
3 cups mixed greens

Snack
Post-Workout Shake (page 85)

Dinner
Chicken Pizza (page 150)

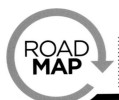

Day 35

PHASE

2

Week

5

29	30	31	32	33	34	35
36	37	38	39	40	41	42
43	44	45	46	47	48	49
50	51	52	53	54	55	56

TODAY'S FOCUS ✓

ACTION: Be prepared.

Get focused for the week. Plan ahead through the next 24 hours and even through the next week. Don't forget about your journal: Continue the habit of writing out your meals a day ahead, as well as when you'll do your workouts. Cook food ahead of time so it's easily accessible in your fridge and ready to go when it's time to prepare meals.

WORKOUT 🏃

DAY OFF: Active Recovery

or, if you want more structure, hit the optional 20-minute interval workout. Go for a walk or a hike or do something active you enjoy, as long as it's not too taxing. Or take the day completely off and relax!

MENU PLAN 🍴

Take supplements: 1 to 2 grams omega-3s, multivitamin, and 1,000 IU vitamin D

Plus 1 serving of Greens+

Breakfast

Smoothie: *1 cup Greek yogurt, 1 cup fresh fruit, and ½ cup 100% orange or grapefruit juice*

Snack

2 tablespoons almond butter
10 celery sticks

Lunch

Asian Chicken Salad (page 94) and Sesame Dressing (page 95)

Snack

Post-Workout Shake (page 85)

Dinner

5 ounces cooked salmon
¾ cup cooked quinoa (cooked in chicken broth instead of water for extra flavor)
Side Salad (page 83) with 1 tablespoon Homemade Vinaigrette (page 151)

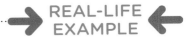
Energy to Spare

AMY NOLAND > dropped four sizes

Every Mother's Day, our church's primary leaders ask the kids "What is your mom's favorite thing to do?" Two years in a row, my kids' response was "Lay in bed and watch TV." I remember after the second year in a row of this response (from both my children), I was mortified and humiliated. After we got home from church, I remember crying to my husband and saying, "Is this how our kids are going to remember me—a couch potato who can't even get up and do anything?"

I didn't know how that had happened, considering I was very active with them when they were little, but maybe that's because I had to be. Two three-year-olds running away from you in opposite directions will make you actively get up and move! But all that changed and I had sunk into being so lethargic. I had no energy. I would get up and get them off to school, and then return to bed and the TV where I'd remain sometimes until they came home from school. It's embarrassing for me to admit that even now.

When I started using the Drop Two Sizes principles, I was 126 pounds and a size 10. Having a set workout plan and nutrition to follow was exactly what I needed. Strength training and lifting heavy weights transformed my body. I dropped four sizes to a size 2, but my weight only dropped 5 pounds because I built lean body mass, completely transforming my body.

I always feel energized and better after I work out. I'm happier! I'm active, fit, and have energy to spare!

The highlight of my year was doing a mud run with my two children. I was no longer the mom sitting at home on the couch or the bed watching TV—we were all out there doing something active together.

before   *after*

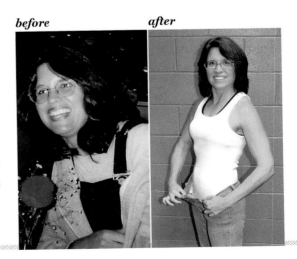

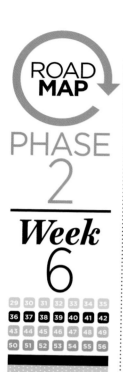

It's Week Six, and you're almost halfway there!

You're also coming up to the next Jeans Check. As we've discussed, this is truly the best measurement of your transformation. Any pair of pants or fitted skirt can serve as your Jeans Check clothing item.

Take a deep breath, and don't get too stressed about trying your goal clothes on again (especially if it didn't go so well the first time). Most of my clients find that by Week Six, they can zip up their jeans (even if it's not pretty or that comfortable!) This week, relax and believe in yourself. If you had any setbacks since the previous Jeans Check, you're overcoming them and following the plan with confidence.

Week Six Plan of Attack:

Use next week's Jeans Check as motivation this week. Dive into your workouts, and really focus on eating right. If you feel the need to splurge more than you should, think of new strategies to say, "No, thank you!" or keep extra healthy snacks on hand when you know you'll crave them most.

Keep sliced cucumber or baby carrots in your fridge for a great, crunchy snack option. Or try one of my favorite go-to snacks: a small bag of coleslaw, rainbow slaw, or broccoli slaw, mixed with tuna, chicken, or other protein—an instantly satisfying salad. You can sprinkle it with olive oil and vinegar for extra flavor and zing.

Week Six Grocery List

PRODUCE

- Apples
- Lemons
- Avocado (1)
- Bell peppers
- Broccoli
- Cucumber
- Eggplant
- Greens, mixed
- Melon
- Potato, white (1 medium)
- Spinach, baby
- Sweet potato (1 large)
- Tomatoes
- Tomatoes, cherry
- Zucchini

DAIRY & EGGS

- Eggs
- Goat cheese
- Greek yogurt, 2% (plain)
- Milk, 2% (cow, soy, or almond)

BAKERY

- Ezekiel bread
- Ezekiel tortillas

MEAT, DELI & SEAFOOD

- Chicken breasts, boneless, skinless (1¼ pounds)
- Flank steak
- Salmon, wild-caught (6 ounces)
- Shrimp
- Tilapia
- Tuna steak

GROCERY & PANTRY

- Almond butter
- Almonds, raw
- Brown rice
- Chickpeas
- Oatmeal (rolled oats)
- Olives
- Peanut butter, natural
- Quinoa
- Raisins
- Salsa
- Whey protein powder

FROZEN

- Berries

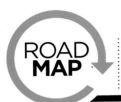

ROAD MAP

PHASE 2

Week 6

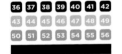

29	30	31	32	33	34	35
36	**37**	**38**	**39**	**40**	**41**	**42**
43	44	45	46	47	48	49
50	51	52	53	54	55	56

Day 36

TODAY'S FOCUS ✓

Checkpoint: **Brake Check**

We talked about this at the end of Week Two. Pay attention to when you start feeling negative about yourself, tend to skip workouts, or rationalize a splurge that wasn't on the plan. Staying mindful of these roadblocks will help you overcome them in the future and gain a greater awareness of what it takes to succeed.

WORKOUT

PHASE 2: STRENGTH 2

MENU PLAN 🍴

Take supplements: 1 to 2 grams omega-3s, multivitamin, and 1,000 IU vitamin D

Plus 1 serving of Greens+

Breakfast

1 cup cooked oatmeal (made with 1 cup fat-free milk)
1 tablespoon raisins
1 tablespoon chopped raw almonds

Snack

¼ cup raw almonds

Lunch

4 ounces grilled chicken breast
1 slice Ezekiel bread topped with 1 ounce goat cheese and sliced tomato

Snack

Post-Workout Shake (page 85)

Dinner

4 ounces grilled tuna steak over a bed of steamed spinach (top with freshly squeezed lemon juice, salt, and pepper to taste)
Side Salad (page 83) with 1 tablespoon Homemade Vinaigrette (page 151)

Day 37

TODAY'S FOCUS

ACTION: What is your "Why"?
This is a good time to revisit
your mission statement. If you
haven't already memorized it,
then memorize it today—and say
it out loud in front of a mirror—
so that you can really use it
over the next 6 weeks. Write
or print it out on a small piece
of paper and tack it above
your desk or on your fridge,
or put it in your wallet as a
constant reminder of your goal.

WORKOUT

DAY OFF: Active Recovery,
optional 20-minute interval
workout, or repeat this week's
metabolic workout.

MENU PLAN

*Take supplements: 1 to 2 grams omega-3s,
multivitamin, and 1,000 IU vitamin D*
Plus 1 serving of Greens+

Breakfast
Breakfast Wrap (page 112)

Snack
*1 apple
1 tablespoon natural peanut butter*

Lunch
Chopped Salad with Shrimp: *3 ounces
cooked shrimp, 3 cups mixed greens,
½ cup chopped tomatoes, ½ cup chopped
cucumber, ¼ cup black olives, ¼ cup
chickpeas, 1 tablespoon olive oil, and
lemon juice to taste*

Snack
Post-Workout Shake (page 85)

Dinner
*6 ounces wild-caught salmon
(skin removed), roasted**
2 cups steamed or roasted broccoli
¾ cup cooked quinoa

**Brush with mustard and roast at 400°F for
20 minutes.*

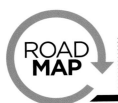

ROAD MAP

Day 38

PHASE

2

Week

6

29	30	31	32	33	34	35
36	37	38	39	40	41	42
43	44	45	46	47	48	49
50	51	52	53	54	55	56

TODAY'S FOCUS ✅

Checkpoint: **Water Check**

Are you drinking enough water? Throughout the challenge, you should consume at least 64 ounces (8 glasses) of water every day. If you have lost track and aren't drinking enough, come up with a strategy today to figure out how you can ramp up your liquids. Maybe it's keeping a pretty glass pitcher in the fridge with lemon slices, or leaving a water bottle on your desk at work.

WORKOUT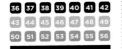

PHASE 2: STRENGTH 1

MENU PLAN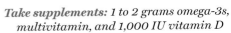

Take supplements: 1 to 2 grams omega-3s, multivitamin, and 1,000 IU vitamin D

Plus 1 serving of Greens+

Breakfast

1 cup cooked oatmeal
 (made with 1 cup fat-free milk)
1 tablespoon raisins
1 tablespoon chopped raw almonds

Snack

¼ cup raw almonds

Lunch

Chicken and Avocado Salad (page 92)

Snack

Post-Workout Shake (page 85)

Dinner

4 ounces grilled shrimp or tilapia
¾ cup cooked brown rice
1 cup cherry tomatoes topped with
 1 tablespoon Homemade Vinaigrette
 (page 151)

Day 39

TODAY'S FOCUS

ACTION: Think ahead.
Pencil in what you are planning to eat over the next 24 hours. In order to be successful, you have to think ahead and not leave anything to chance.

WORKOUT

DAY OFF: Active Recovery
or complete day of rest.

MENU PLAN

Take supplements: 1 to 2 grams omega-3s, multivitamin, and 1,000 IU vitamin D
Plus 1 serving of Greens+

Breakfast
Breakfast Wrap (page 112)

Snack
1 apple
1 cup 2% Greek yogurt topped with a drizzle of honey

Lunch
4 ounces grilled chicken breast
1 slice Ezekiel bread topped with 1 ounce goat cheese and sliced tomato

Snack
Post-Workout Shake (page 85)

Dinner
1 large baked sweet potato topped with 1 cup cooked broccoli and 2 tablespoons 2% Greek yogurt
Side Salad (page 83) with 1 tablespoon Homemade Vinaigrette (page 151)

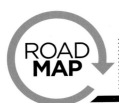

ROAD MAP

PHASE 2

Week 6

29	30	31	32	33	34	35
36	37	38	39	40	41	42
43	44	45	46	47	48	49
50	51	52	53	54	55	56

Day 40

TODAY'S FOCUS ✓

ACTION: Stick to it.

"Stick to it and get through it." Change is tough, but you are tougher! Remember the commitment you made to yourself on Day 1, and use that resolve to get through any uncomfortable situations today.

WORKOUT

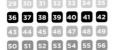

PHASE 2: STRENGTH 2

MENU PLAN 🍴

Take supplements: 1 to 2 grams omega-3s, multivitamin, and 1,000 IU vitamin D

Plus 1 serving of Greens+

Breakfast
1 slice Ezekiel bread, toasted
2 tablespoons natural peanut butter

Snack
1 apple
10 raw almonds

Lunch
Chopped Salad with Shrimp (page 161)

Snack
Post-Workout Shake (page 85)

Dinner
5 ounces grilled chicken breast
1 medium potato, chopped and roasted with 2 teaspoons olive oil
Side Salad (page 83) with 1 tablespoon Homemade Vinaigrette (page 151)

Day 41

TODAY'S FOCUS

Checkpoint: **Sleep Check**

Have you been going to bed at the same time each night and waking up at the same time each morning? Are you making your room as dark as possible and staying off the computer and TV for at least an hour before bedtime? Sleep is when your body recovers and regenerates. If you aren't getting enough sleep, it will be hard to lose fat. Try doing something relaxing before bed, such as reading a book or magazine, or doing a few minutes of deep breathing.

WORKOUT

PHASE 2: COMPLEX METABOLIC

MENU PLAN

Take supplements: 1 to 2 grams omega-3s, multivitamin, and 1,000 IU vitamin D
Plus 1 serving of Greens+

Breakfast

*1 cup cooked oatmeal
    (made with 1 cup fat-free milk)*
1 tablespoon raisins
1 tablespoon chopped raw almonds

Snack

1 apple
*1 cup 2% Greek yogurt topped
    with a drizzle of honey*

Lunch

*2 slices Ezekiel bread with 2 tablespoons
    natural peanut butter*

Snack

Post-Workout Shake (page 85)

Dinner

5 ounces grilled flank steak
*2 cups roasted or grilled vegetables
    (zucchini, eggplant, bell pepper)*

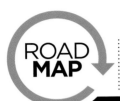

Day 42

PHASE 2

Week 6

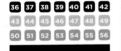

29	30	31	32	33	34	35
36	37	38	39	40	41	42
43	44	45	46	47	48	49
50	51	52	53	54	55	56

TODAY'S FOCUS ⊘

ACTION: Reflect.
Take today to reflect on the last 6 weeks. What is working really well for you? What can you still improve on? Get focused as you head into the final weeks of your journey!

WORKOUT

DAY OFF: Active Recovery or complete day of rest.

MENU PLAN ▮▮

Take supplements: 1 to 2 grams omega-3s, multivitamin, and 1,000 IU vitamin D
Plus 1 serving of Greens+

Breakfast
1 slice Ezekiel bread
2 tablespoons almond butter

Snack
1 cup 2% Greek yogurt
½ cup diced melon or other fresh fruit

Lunch
Chicken and Avocado Salad (page 92)

Snack
Post-Workout Shake (page 85)

Dinner
4 ounces grilled shrimp or tilapia
1 cup cooked zucchini
1 cup cooked quinoa

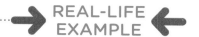
Committed to Real Change

KATHLEE COLEMAN > dropped two sizes in 8 weeks

When I started learning the Drop Two Sizes principles, I had already lost 60 pounds with a different weight loss program. While that was great, I was focused only on losing weight, not on replacing fat with muscle. My body hadn't changed in quite a while—I was at a stagnant point, and I was a bit skeptical that I could lose even one jean size in 8 weeks, much less two. However, I went into the challenge with a positive attitude, and a resolve to give it 100 percent in every way. I tried on a pair of size 12 jeans that fit well, so I bought an 8. They weren't even close to buttoning! But I was determined to do what it took to get into them.

I had to make certain commitments to myself and to others in order to do it. I had to commit to at least four workouts a week. I put them on my calendar as appointments that I scheduled other events around—there was no way I was going to miss a workout! I planned my meals for the week, helping me to shop smart when I went to the grocery story and to stick to my plan.

Three weeks into the challenge, the size 8s actually buttoned. They weren't comfortable and didn't look great, but they buttoned. I was thrilled and motivated! At week 6, the jeans fit well enough to wear out, and by week 8 they fit me like a glove. I've actually gained ten pounds since joining the gym—I didn't lose a pound during the challenge! Who would have guessed I'd gain weight, but wear jeans that are two sizes smaller? Rachel has inspired me to reach beyond what I thought was possible and given me the confidence to set new goals and consider things I never would have before!

before   *after*

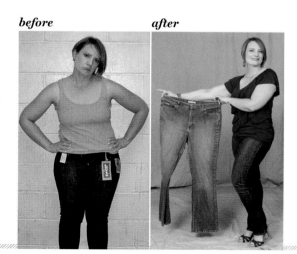

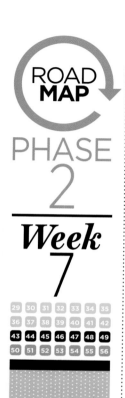

ROAD MAP

PHASE 2

Week 7

29	30	31	32	33	34	35
36	37	38	39	40	41	42
43	**44**	**45**	**46**	**47**	**48**	**49**
50	51	52	53	54	55	56

Welcome to Week Seven, over halfway there!

You've reached a big milestone and passed the half-way point of your journey. Congrats! Along the way you may have encountered a few obstacles that deterred you. But, as with any road trip, even if you took a detour or had to pull off the highway, you got right back on the road toward your destination.

Remember, you've embarked on a challenge, not a diet. The road that will get you from Point A to Point B is not always quick or easy. But this time, you'll reach Point B, or that glorious moment when you slide on your clothes and realize you look and feel fabulous—and you'll stay that way for the rest of your life! Keep reminding yourself what lies ahead and use it to motivate and inspire you to keep going.

Week Seven
Plan of Attack:

Refocus. Let's step on that accelerator as you head toward your goal. If you've been consistently following the road map, you may find that at this week's Jeans Check, your clothes already fit! Many clients have dropped two sizes in just 6 to 8 weeks.

If you've arrived at your destination early, take a moment to congratulate yourself, and let yourself enjoy that feeling of accomplishment. You may decide to continue on the next 6 weeks to see how truly fit and fabulous you can get, or you may decide to incorporate the following road map into your lifestyle to maintain your current figure.

Either way, there are plenty of great workouts and actions ahead that will help you stick to your goal.

Week Seven Grocery List

PRODUCE

- Apples
- Bananas
- Lemons
- Pineapple
- Bell peppers
- Broccoli
- Carrots, baby
- Celery
- Cucumber
- Green beans
- Greens, mixed
- Mushrooms
- Potato, white (1 medium)
- Spinach, baby
- Sweet potato (1 medium)
- Tomatoes
- Basil
- Garlic
- Hummus

DAIRY & EGGS

- Cheese, mozzarella, shredded
- Cottage cheese, low-fat
- Eggs
- Goat cheese
- Greek yogurt, 2% (plain)
- Milk, 2% (cow, soy, or almond)

BAKERY

- Ezekiel bread
- Ezekiel English muffins
- Ezekiel tortillas

MEAT, DELI & SEAFOOD

- Chicken breasts, boneless, skinless (1¾ pounds)
- Chicken thighs, boneless, skinless (6 ounces)
- Pork tenderloin (about ¾ pound)
- Salmon, wild-caught (about ¾ pound)
- Shrimp (about ½ pound)

GROCERY & PANTRY

- Almond butter
- Barbecue sauce
- Brown rice
- Chickpeas
- Flax seeds, ground
- Kashi Go Lean cereal
- Muir Glen Organic Marinara Sauce
- Olives
- Pasta, whole grain
- Quinoa
- Whey protein powder

FROZEN

- Berries

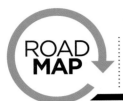

Day 43

PHASE

2

Week

7

29	30	31	32	33	34	35
36	37	38	39	40	41	42
43	**44**	**45**	**46**	**47**	**48**	**49**
50	51	52	53	54	55	56

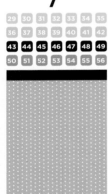

TODAY'S FOCUS ✓

Checkpoint: **Jeans Check**

Try your clothes on today! By now you should notice a fairly dramatic difference in the way your clothes fit compared to Week One. If they still don't quite fit, remember you still have 6 more weeks to hit your goal!

WORKOUT

PHASE 2: STRENGTH 1

MENU PLAN

Take supplements: 1 to 2 grams omega-3s, multivitamin, and 1,000 IU vitamin D
Plus 1 serving of Greens+

Breakfast
1 Ezekiel English muffin
2 tablespoons almond butter

Snack
1 hard-cooked egg
1 piece fruit

Lunch
Chicken Salad Wrap* (Day 44)

*Make a double batch of the chicken salad mixture for lunch on Day 46.

Snack
Post-Workout Shake (page 85)

Dinner
5 ounces grilled wild-caught salmon (or any other favorite fish)
Sweet Potato Fries: *1 medium sweet potato (cut into fries), drizzled with 2 teaspoons olive oil, seasoned with salt and pepper, and roasted at 400°F for 30 to 40 minutes*
Side Salad (page 83) with 1 tablespoon Homemade Vinaigrette (page 151)

Day 44

TODAY'S FOCUS

ACTION: Track your habits.
Have you been filling out your journal? If not, start to track everything again. In 2 weeks you will have another Splurge Check, and if you're not tracking your habits, you won't know where you need to improve, and where you can allow yourself a bit more leeway. It's important to know where you stand.

WORKOUT

DAY OFF: Active Recovery, optional 20-minute interval workout, or repeat the metabolic workout from this week.

MENU PLAN

Take supplements: 1 to 2 grams omega-3s, multivitamin, and 1,000 IU vitamin D
Plus 1 serving of Greens+

Breakfast
1 cup low-fat cottage cheese
1 cup fresh fruit
1 tablespoon ground flax seeds

Snack
¼ cup hummus
10 baby carrots

Lunch
Chopped Salad with Shrimp (page 161)

Snack
Post-Workout Shake (page 85)

Dinner
Chicken Parmesan: *5 ounces cooked chicken breast topped with ½ cup marinara sauce (Muir Glen Organic recommended), thinly sliced bell pepper (to taste), and ⅓ cup shredded mozzarella cheese**

*Place under the broiler for 2 to 3 minutes to melt the cheese.

Side Salad (page 83) with 1 tablespoon Homemade Vinaigrette (page 151)

Chicken Salad Wrap

3 ounces cooked chicken breast, shredded or diced

Chopped celery, to taste

1 tablespoon 2% Greek yogurt

1 teaspoon prepared mustard

Fresh herbs

1 Ezekiel tortilla

1 cup baby spinach

Mix the chicken, celery, yogurt, mustard, and herbs, and wrap in the tortilla. Serve with baby spinach on the side. You can make a double batch of this salad and keep it in the fridge for a snack or lunch the same week.

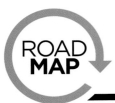

Day 45

PHASE 2

Week 7

29	30	31	32	33	34	35
36	37	38	39	40	41	42
43	**44**	**45**	**46**	**47**	**48**	**49**
50	51	52	53	54	55	56

TODAY'S FOCUS ☑

Checkpoint: **Veggie Check**
This week you should bump up to at least six servings of veggies per day. Remember that one serving equals 1 cup or the size of your fist. You can do it! Explore and try a new veggie today, maybe kale or eggplant. Check out the recipe section to get some ideas.

WORKOUT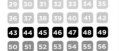

PHASE 2: STRENGTH 2

MENU PLAN 🍴

Take supplements: 1 to 2 grams omega-3s, multivitamin, and 1,000 IU vitamin D
Plus 1 serving of Greens+

Breakfast
1 egg + 3 egg whites in an omelet with 1 cup spinach and a handful of mushrooms

Snack
1 hard-cooked egg
1 piece fruit

Lunch
Hummus and Veggie Wrap: *1 Ezekiel tortilla filled with ¼ cup hummus and 1 cup vegetables*

Snack
Post-Workout Shake (page 85)

Dinner
6 ounces cooked boneless, skinless chicken thighs*
1 cup cooked quinoa
1 cup steamed green beans drizzled with 2 teaspoons olive oil and a sprinkle of sea salt

*Brush with barbecue sauce and grill or roast.

Day 46

TODAY'S FOCUS

Checkpoint: **Posture Check**
Today, stand up tall, keeping your core engaged and your shoulders pulled down and back. Having excellent posture gives you the confidence to tackle the day. You know what you want and how you will get it.

WORKOUT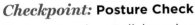

DAY OFF: Active Recovery
or complete day of rest.

MENU PLAN

Take supplements: 1 to 2 grams omega-3s, multivitamin, and 1,000 IU vitamin D
Plus 1 serving of Greens+

Breakfast
1 cup Kashi Go Lean cereal
¾ cup fat-free milk
½ banana, sliced

Snack
¼ cup hummus
10 baby carrots

Lunch
1 Chicken Salad Wrap (page 171)
1 cup cubed pineapple or other fresh fruit

Snack
Post-Workout Shake (page 85)

Dinner
5 ounces grilled or roasted pork tenderloin
2 cups broccoli roasted with 2 teaspoons extra virgin olive oil
¾ cup cooked brown rice

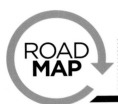

ROAD MAP

Day 47

PHASE

2

Week

7

29	30	31	32	33	34	35
36	37	38	39	40	41	42
43	**44**	**45**	**46**	**47**	**48**	**49**
50	51	52	53	54	55	56

TODAY'S FOCUS ✓

ACTION: Stick to your commitment.
Remember your three favorite words: "No, thank you."
Heading into the weekend, remind yourself that only you can stick to your commitment and have control over your body. Anything that doesn't fit in that plan should be told, "No, thank you!"

WORKOUT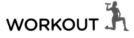

PHASE 2: STRENGTH 1

MENU PLAN 🍴

Take supplements: 1 to 2 grams omega-3s, multivitamin, and 1,000 IU vitamin D
Plus 1 serving of Greens+

Breakfast
1 cup Kashi Go Lean cereal
¾ cup 2% milk
½ banana, sliced

Snack
¼ cup hummus
10 baby carrots

Lunch
Chopped Salad with Shrimp (page 161)
1 piece fresh fruit

Snack
Post-Workout Shake (page 85)

Dinner
Pesto Salmon: *5 ounces wild-caught salmon (skin removed), roasted. Brush the salmon with a thin layer of Pesto (see opposite) and roast at 400°F for 20 minutes.**
2 cups steamed green beans

*Save extra Pesto for dinner on Day 49.

Day 48

TODAY'S FOCUS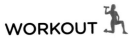

ACTION: Don't forget the little things.

They can make a big difference: Consistently taking your omega-3s and your multivitamin are two great examples. Make sure you continue to make both of these part of your regimen every single day.

WORKOUT

PHASE 2: TIMED METABOLIC

MENU PLAN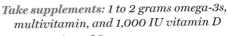

Take supplements: 1 to 2 grams omega-3s, multivitamin, and 1,000 IU vitamin D
Plus 1 serving of Greens+

Breakfast
1 Ezekiel English muffin
2 tablespoons almond butter

Snack
¼ cup hummus
10 baby carrots

Lunch
4 ounces grilled chicken breast
1 slice Ezekiel bread topped with 1 ounce goat cheese and sliced tomato
1 apple

Snack
Post-Workout Shake (page 85)

Dinner
Chicken Parmesan (page 171)
1 cup cooked whole grain pasta

Pesto

1 bunch fresh basil
1 clove garlic
1 pinch each salt and pepper
½ cup extra virgin olive oil

Combine the basil, garlic, salt, and pepper in a blender. Turn the machine on and drizzle in just enough extra virgin olive oil to make a paste.

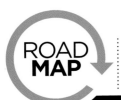

ROAD MAP

PHASE 2

Week 7

29	30	31	32	33	34	35
36	37	38	39	40	41	42
43	**44**	**45**	**46**	**47**	**48**	**49**
50	51	52	53	54	55	56

Day 49

TODAY'S FOCUS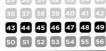

ACTION: Reflect, focus, and plan ahead.

Wow! You have come so far! You've already completed 7 weeks in your journey, and you've built many positive, healthy habits along the way. Reflect on the last 7 weeks. What is working for you? What do you need to improve? Take time today to plan ahead for the next week.

WORKOUT

DAY OFF: Active Recovery or complete day of rest.

MENU PLAN

Take supplements: 1 to 2 grams omega-3s, multivitamin, and 1,000 IU vitamin D
Plus 1 serving of Greens+

Breakfast
1 cup Kashi Go Lean cereal
¾ cup 2% milk
½ banana, sliced

Snack
1 hard-cooked egg
1 piece fruit

Lunch
Grilled Chicken Salad (page 104)

Snack
Post-Workout Shake (page 85)

Dinner
5 ounces grilled or roasted pork tenderloin
Pesto Smashed Potatoes: *Boil 1 medium potato (diced) until tender; mash with 1 tablespoon Pesto (page 175)*

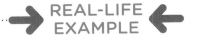
An Athlete Within

MICHELLE MUDROW > dropped from a size 28 to a size 10

From an early age I adopted unhealthy eating habits. I wasn't physically active other than playing outside with friends. I let the negative voices I heard from society and from those around me keep me in my fat cage for almost 30 years. It affected my daily decisions and my relationships. I settled for less than I wanted or deserved . . . a lot. I was told, "Fat girls don't go to the gym," and I believed it.

In 2007 I was at my absolute worst. I had hit rock bottom, and my weight had sky-rocketed to an all-time high of 275 pounds. I was trapped in an abusive marriage, surviving only with the help of anti-depressants, and physically unable to walk around my block comfortably. One day I saw an adver-tisement on TV for a lap-band procedure, and I actually wrote down the number. It clicked: if I was willing to invest that kind of money into a surgery, why wasn't I willing to invest that same money into myself?

Embarrassed and ashamed (but oh so determined), I marched into my local gym the week before Christmas and asked for a trainer. I discovered I had a natural knack

for lifting and I really enjoyed it. Being strong physically made me stronger in other areas of my life, too. I not only dropped in size, I also lost years of emotional baggage.

With the plan in Drop Two Sizes, I lost 115 pounds, 20 percent of my body fat, and about 90 inches. My jeans went from a size 28 to a size 10. I am now certified as a trainer and have a passion for helping other women discover what it means to be "strong." I transformed my body and my life dramatically because of it. That feels *really* good to say!

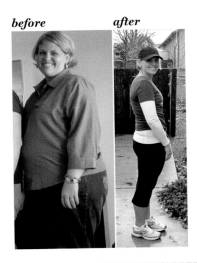

before   *after*

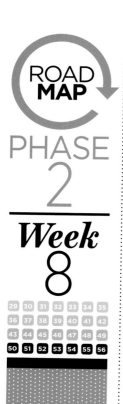

ROAD MAP

PHASE 2

Week 8

It's Week Eight.

You're now 8 weeks into this program. You've been following my nutrition recommendations, doing the training programs, and building a new and dynamic lifestyle for yourself. You should start to feel like you own this plan! As your clothes continue to fit better and you feel better wearing them, your confidence should be growing too.

Your friends and family are probably starting to notice how much you have changed and may have complimented you on your progress so far. Maybe you have even started to inspire others to join the challenge too and drop two sizes.

Remember that fit chicks of a feather flock together! Having a friend to support you as you continue your journey, or even join you, can make all the difference.

Week Eight Plan of Attack:

Make it stick! I mentioned that it usually takes around 30 days to successfully build habits. Now, as you finish the second 30 days, the goal is to really own these habits and make them yours for the long term. These are *your* Menu Plans, *your* workouts, and those are *your* hot outfits waiting for you in your closet!

Continue doing whatever works for you to stick to the plan. Make dates with a friend to work out together and keep each other accountable. Swap your favorite clothes to keep each other excited and motivated. Keep track of all your progress in your journal. Remind yourself how much you rock!

Week Eight Grocery List

PRODUCE

- Apples
- Bananas
- Lemons
- Melon or pineapple
- Orange
- Strawberries
- Asparagus
- Avocado (1)
- Beets
- Bell peppers (red)
- Broccoli
- Celery
- Cucumber
- Greens, mixed
- Onion, red
- Spinach, baby
- Sweet potato (1 small)
- Tomato

DAIRY & EGGS

- Cheese, shredded
- Cheese, string
- Cottage cheese, low-fat
- Eggs
- Feta cheese, crumbled
- Milk, 2% (cow, soy, or almond)

BAKERY

- Ezekiel tortilla

FROZEN

- Berries
- Van's Whole Grain Waffles

MEAT, DELI & SEAFOOD

- Chicken breasts, boneless, skinless (about ¾ pound)
- Pork tenderloin (about ¼ pound)
- Salmon, wild-caught (¾ pound)
- Tilapia (about ⅓ pound)
- Turkey breast, ground

GROCERY & PANTRY

- Ak-mak crackers
- Almond butter
- Almonds, raw
- Beans, black, canned
- Beans, red kidney, canned (15 ounces)
- Beans, pinto, canned (15 ounces)
- Beer, dark
- Broth, low-sodium chicken
- Brown rice
- Cumin, ground
- Kashi Go Lean cereal
- Kashi Granola Bars
- Lara Bar
- Salmon (canned)
- Salsa
- Tomatoes, crushed (3 cans, 28 ounces each)
- Whey protein powder

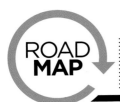

Day 50

PHASE
2

Week
8

29	30	31	32	33	34	35
36	37	38	39	40	41	42
43	44	45	46	47	48	49
50	**51**	**52**	**53**	**54**	**55**	**56**

TODAY'S FOCUS ☑

ACTION: Visualize.

Start your week off on the right foot. Take today to refocus if you need to and think about how close you are to finishing this challenge. Throughout your workout, visualize yourself rocking your favorite outfit, and looking fabulous!

WORKOUT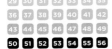

PHASE 2: STRENGTH 2

MENU PLAN 🍴

Take supplements: 1 to 2 grams omega-3s, multivitamin, and 1,000 IU vitamin D
Plus 1 serving of Greens+

Breakfast
1 whole grain waffle (Van's brand recommended) topped with 2 tablespoons almond butter, ½ cup sliced strawberries, and a drizzle of honey

Snack
1 cup low-fat cottage cheese
1 cup diced melon or pineapple

Lunch
Beet Salad (page 112)
1 banana

Snack
Post-Workout Shake (page 85)

Dinner
1 serving Turkey Chili* (see opposite)

*Save a serving for dinner on Day 52. Store the remaining chili in the freezer for an upcoming week.

Day 51

TODAY'S FOCUS ✅

ACTION: Are you eating enough?
How hungry are you? Are you dieting too hard? If you find yourself bingeing during your splurges instead of simply enjoying a treat and the experience surrounding it, then you probably aren't eating enough the rest of the week. Bump up your good fats including avocado, olive oil, nuts, or coconut milk. Have a source of good fats with each meal.

WORKOUT 🏃

DAY OFF: Active Recovery, optional 20-minute interval workout, or repeat metabolic workout from this week.

MENU PLAN 🍴

Take supplements: 1 to 2 grams omega-3s, multivitamin, and 1,000 IU vitamin D
Plus 1 serving of Greens+

Breakfast

Omelet Cup: *1 egg + 1 egg white scrambled with ¼ cup shredded cheese in a coffee cup. Microwave on high for 60 seconds.*
1 cup fresh fruit

Snack

1 string cheese
1 apple

Lunch

3 ounces canned salmon mixed with ½ cup chopped celery, 1 tablespoon olive oil mayonnaise, and Dijon mustard to taste
3 cups mixed greens
5 ak-mak or RyKrisp crackers
1 apple

Snack

Post-Workout Shake (page 85)

Dinner

6 ounces wild-caught salmon (skin removed), roasted*
2 cups steamed or roasted broccoli
¾ cup cooked brown rice

*Brush with mustard and roast at 400°F for 20 minutes.

Turkey Chili

1 tablespoon canola oil

1 pound ground turkey breast

1 medium red onion, diced

1 red bell pepper, diced

½ teaspoon kosher salt

½ cup low-sodium chicken broth or water

4 ounces dark beer

3 cans (28 ounces each) crushed tomatoes

1 teaspoon ground cumin

2 tablespoons chili powder or to taste

1 can (15 ounces) pinto beans, rinsed and drained

1 can (15 ounces) red kidney beans, rinsed and drained

In a large pot or Dutch oven over medium heat, heat the oil. Add the turkey and cook until browned stirring frequently,

>> Cont'd on page 183

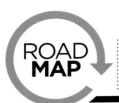

Day 52

PHASE
2

Week
8

29	30	31	32	33	34	35
36	37	38	39	40	41	42
43	44	45	46	47	48	49
50	**51**	**52**	**53**	**54**	**55**	**56**

TODAY'S FOCUS

ACTION: Time to cut the cheese?
What are you leaning on too much? Nuts? Nut butter? Cheese? Are you finding yourself grabbing one of these more than once per day at the most? If your results seem to have reached a plateau, it may be time to cut back and find a different snack option.

WORKOUT

PHASE 2: STRENGTH 1

MENU PLAN

Take supplements: 1 to 2 grams omega-3s, multivitamin, and 1,000 IU vitamin D
Plus 1 serving of Greens+

Breakfast
1 cup Kashi Go Lean cereal
¾ cup 2% milk
½ banana, sliced

Snack
¼ cup raw almonds

Lunch
Rice Bowl (page 102)

Snack
Post-Workout Shake (page 85)

Dinner
1 serving Turkey Chili (page 181)
3 cups mixed greens topped with 2 teaspoons extra virgin olive oil and lemon juice

Day 53

TODAY'S FOCUS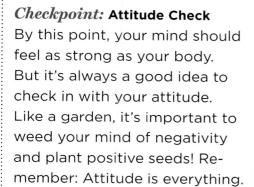

Checkpoint: **Attitude Check**

By this point, your mind should feel as strong as your body. But it's always a good idea to check in with your attitude. Like a garden, it's important to weed your mind of negativity and plant positive seeds! Remember: Attitude is everything.

WORKOUT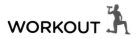

DAY OFF: **Active Recovery**
or complete day of rest.

MENU PLAN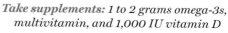

Take supplements: 1 to 2 grams omega-3s, multivitamin, and 1,000 IU vitamin D
Plus 1 serving of Greens+

Breakfast
Omelet Cup (page 181)
1 cup fresh fruit

Snack
1 cup low-fat cottage cheese
½ cup diced melon or pineapple

Lunch
Beet Salad (page 112)
1 banana

Snack
Post-Workout Shake (page 85)

Dinner
4 ounces roasted or grilled pork tenderloin
1 small baked sweet potato
2 cups cooked asparagus

Turkey Chili

>> Cont'd from page 181

Add the onion and pepper and cook, stirring frequently, for 3 to 5 minutes, or until tender. Stir in the salt. Stir in the broth, beer, and tomatoes. Add the cumin and chili powder and stir well to combine; stir in the beans. Bring to a simmer and cook, uncovered, for 25 minutes, stirring occasionally. Makes 8 servings.

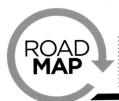
Day 54

ROAD MAP

PHASE

2

Week

8

29	30	31	32	33	34	35
36	37	38	39	40	41	42
43	44	45	46	47	48	49
50	**51**	**52**	**53**	**54**	**55**	**56**

TODAY'S FOCUS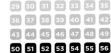

ACTION: Push yourself today.
Today you will do your Phase Two, Strength 2 program one last time. By now you know the exercises. Really push yourself to lift more weight, do all of the sets, and finish strong! You have permission to chill out this upcoming weekend. Give yourself some time to truly decompress, do something indulgent for yourself, and celebrate how far you have come. Take a deep breath and enjoy!

WORKOUT

PHASE 2: STRENGTH 2

MENU PLAN

Take supplements: 1 to 2 grams omega-3s, multivitamin, and 1,000 IU vitamin D
Plus 1 serving of Greens+

Breakfast
1 cup Kashi Go Lean cereal
¾ cup 2% milk
½ banana, sliced

Snack
Kashi Granola Bar

Lunch
3 ounces canned salmon mixed with ½ cup chopped celery, 1 tablespoon olive oil mayonnaise, and Dijon mustard to taste
3 cups mixed greens
1 orange

Snack
Post-Workout Shake (page 85)

Dinner
Chicken Burrito (page 94)

Day 55

TODAY'S FOCUS

Checkpoint: **De-Stress Check**
Have you been taking 10 minutes each day to de-stress? If not, start back up again today. Taking the time to de-stress is an important part of the program and part of your lifetime road map to success. Don't skip it!

WORKOUT

PHASE 2: COMPLEX METABOLIC

MENU PLAN

Take supplements: 1 to 2 grams omega-3s, multivitamin, and 1,000 IU vitamin D
Plus 1 serving of Greens+

Breakfast
1 whole grain waffle (Van's brand recommended) topped with 2 tablespoons almond butter, ½ cup sliced strawberries, and a drizzle of honey

Snack
1 Lara Bar

Lunch
Rice Bowl (page 102)

Snack
Post-Workout Shake (page 85)

Dinner
6 ounces wild-caught salmon (skin removed), roasted*
2 cups broccoli roasted with 2 teaspoons olive oil

*Brush with mustard and roast at 400°F for 20 minutes.

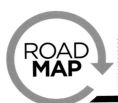

Day 56

PHASE
2

Week
8

29	30	31	32	33	34	35
36	37	38	39	40	41	42
43	44	45	46	47	48	49
50	**51**	**52**	**53**	**54**	**55**	**56**

TODAY'S FOCUS ✅

ACTION: Plan the next 24 hours.
Get focused for the following
week—and the final leg of
the plan. Plan your meals and
workout times for the next
24 hours and through the
next week.

WORKOUT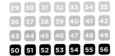

DAY OFF: Active Recovery
or complete day of rest.

MENU PLAN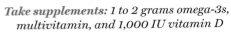

*Take supplements: 1 to 2 grams omega-3s,
multivitamin, and 1,000 IU vitamin D*
Plus 1 serving of Greens+

Breakfast
Omelet Cup (page 181)
1 cup fresh fruit

Snack
1 cup low-fat cottage cheese
1 cup diced melon or pineapple

Lunch
Grilled Tilapia Salad: *3 cups mixed
greens, 1 cup mixed vegetables
(such as cucumber, bell pepper, and
tomato), 5 ounces grilled tilapia, and
2 tablespoons Homemade Vinaigrette
(page 151)*

Snack
Post-Workout Shake (page 85)

Dinner
Chicken Burrito (page 94)

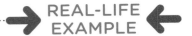
The Power of Goals

ROXANE GRAY > dropped three sizes

I really wanted to enter my thirties in the best shape of my life. My first goal was to complete a half-marathon. But even with all the running, my body didn't transform the way I hoped it would. After the first 4 weeks on the Drop Two Sizes plan, my abs and torso got leaner than from any other workout. I decided to give up running to focus on transforming my body.

I started fitting into clothes that I hadn't seen in 2 years. I got so many compliments when I worked out with my friend and then later at the pool. It's fun to find things to wear again and it's a relief to have that stress gone.

I started training for my first powerlifting competition and became more and more confident in my clothes and in the weight room. I resisted TONS of temptation— and I earned a medal at the competition! I was hooked on my goals! I went to Hawaii and loved being able to wear a bathing suit and not hide from the camera. I thought I had a butt before, but whoa mama, the workouts really lifted my booty.

I decided to train for a bikini competition and I totally rocked it! I feel so empowered that I made the decision to transform myself. I achieved my original goal and then some!

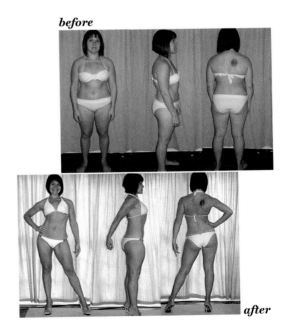

before

after

PHASE THREE

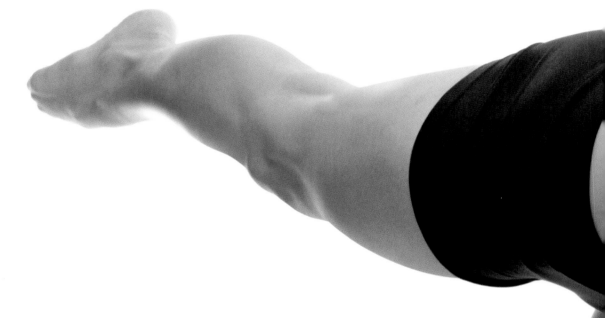

"With *Drop Two Sizes*, even with the workout schedule, I never felt tired or weak. I never felt hungry or craved my favorites (cola and sugar). Planning helped!"

-SHERYL FARLAND, DROPPED TWO SIZES IN 2 WEEKS

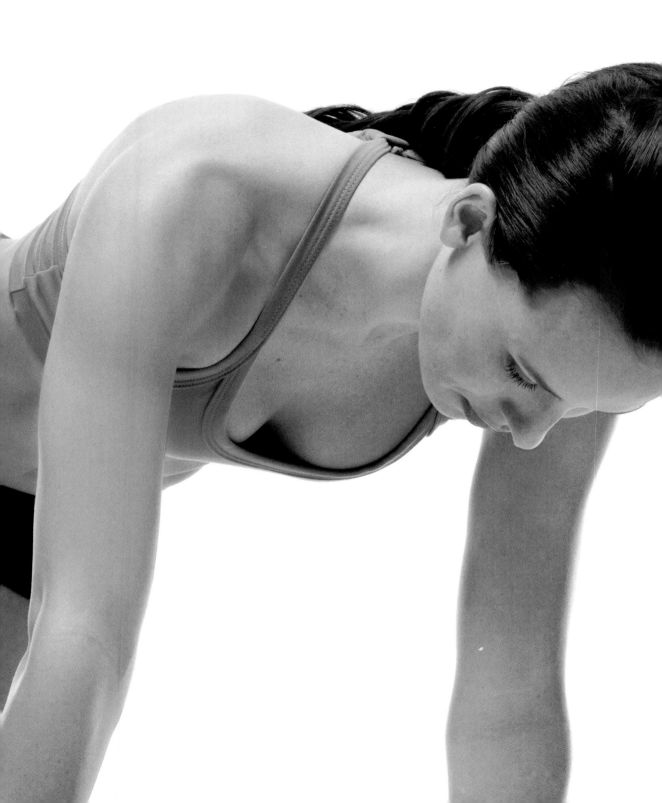

You've come a long way, baby! You've completed 8 weeks of a challenging program, and you may already fit into your jeans or favorite clothes with ease. Continue sticking to the plan—it's working!

PHASE 3:
Road Maps

Read through the following weekly road maps before you get started, and then go through them again each week as you follow the plan. Commit to following the next 30 days of this plan as closely as possible. Get yourself hooked on feeling fit, rather than focusing on trying to reach a number on the scale by the end of the second month.

eating more berries and more green veggies. You'll also no longer eat starchy carbohydrates at dinner during this phase—but you can eat your starches earlier in the day.

By now, your metabolism is revved up and ready to go, and these small tweaks will turbocharge your results!

PHASE 3:
Menu Plan

In this final phase, you want to dial in on real results through your diet as well as your workouts. Using the following menus, you'll up your veggie intake to shoot for 10 servings a day and limit certain fruits, with a focus on

GOALS OF PHASE 3:

→ *Consume 10 servings of vegetables a day.*

→ *Swap out more of your fruits for berries, which are super high in fiber, low in calories, and provide tons of nutrients compared to other fruits.*

→ *Eliminate starchy carbohydrates from your very last meal of the day.*

PHASE 3: **Workouts**

The following is your plan for the next 4 weeks. It's laid out here to make sure you can plan ahead and make time for all the workouts, to achieve the best possible results. Do not add anything, change anything, or skip anything. All you need to do is commit to taking it one day at a time!

	Monday	Tuesday	Wednesday	Thursday	Friday	Saturday	Sunday
Week 9	Day 57 STRENGTH WORKOUT 1	Day 58 DAY OFF: Active Recovery or optional 20-minute interval session	Day 59 STRENGTH WORKOUT 2	Day 60 DAY OFF: Active Recovery	Day 61 STRENGTH WORKOUT 1	Day 62 COUNT-DOWN METABOLIC	Day 63 DAY OFF: Active Recovery
Week 10	Day 64 STRENGTH WORKOUT 2	Day 65 DAY OFF: Active Recovery or optional 20-minute interval session	Day 66 STRENGTH WORKOUT 1	Day 67 DAY OFF: Active Recovery	Day 68 STRENGTH WORKOUT 2	Day 69 COMPLEX METABOLIC	Day 70 DAY OFF: Active Recovery
Week 11	Day 71 STRENGTH WORKOUT 1	Day 72 DAY OFF: Active Recovery or optional 20-minute interval session	Day 73 STRENGTH WORKOUT 2	Day 74 DAY OFF: Active Recovery	Day 75 STRENGTH WORKOUT 1	Day 76 COUNT-DOWN METABOLIC	Day 77 DAY OFF: Active Recovery
Week 12	Day 78 STRENGTH WORKOUT 2	Day 79 DAY OFF: Active Recovery or optional 20-minute interval session	Day 80 STRENGTH WORKOUT 1	Day 81 DAY OFF: Active Recovery	Day 82 STRENGTH WORKOUT 2	Day 83 COMPLEX METABOLIC	Day 84 DAY OFF: Active Recovery

PHASE 3: RAMP

Perform one set of each of the following warmup exercises before you start each workout.

1 **Foam Roller/Self-Myofascial Release Full Body**

2 **Half-Kneeling Hip Flexor Stretch with Rotation and Rear Foot Elevated** (Hold for 30 seconds on each side)

3 **Hip/Thigh Extension** (8 reps on each side, hold for 1 second at the top of each rep)

4 **Elevated Plank Hip External Rotation Knee Raise** (5 reps on each side with a 2-second hold)

5 **Open Half-Kneeling with Thoracic Reach** (5 reps on each side)

6 **Squat to Stand 2** (10 reps)

7 **Inchworm** (10 reps)

8 **Open Half-Kneeling with Ankle Mobilization** (5 reps on each side)

9 **Forward/Back Hop** (10 reps on each side)

10 **Forward/Back Leg Swing** (8 reps on each side)

11 **Lateral Hop** (10 reps on each side)

12 **Cross-in-Front Lunge** (6 reps on each side)

13 **Cross-Body Knee Hug to a Lunge** (15 reps on each side)

RAMP 1: Foam Roller/ Self-Myofascial Release

Hopefully you purchased a foam roller for your home (or a lacrosse ball, which can be used as a massage ball). These tools work great to massage your muscle without having to fork over big bucks for a professional masseuse.

As you go through the RAMP stretches and movements on the following pages, notice where you feel tight—you can use the foam roller or ball to massage that area. Eventually you can work through your entire body. In addition, you can roll out your tensor fascia latae (TFL) and iliotibial (IT) band by lying on your side and rolling the outside of your leg from your hip to your knee. This tends to be a pretty sore spot, but you'll be glad you did it!

Your muscles will probably be tender the first time you roll them out, so don't push through any pain if it becomes excruciating. If it is so painful that you're tensing up, the exercise won't work as designed. Each time you use the foam roller it should feel less uncomfortable. Ideally, you'll want to use the foam roller a few minutes each day.

Use it regularly to avoid injury and feel great after your workouts! Focus on rolling out 3 to 5 areas that feel tight.

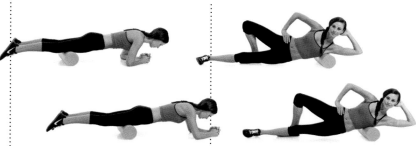

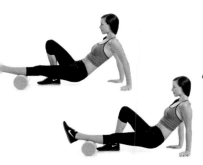

Calves

POSITION: Place your left calf on the roller and support yourself, putting as much weight on the calf as you can. Turn your left leg in and roll so you are massaging the inside of your left calf. Then turn your toe straight up and roll and finish with your toe turned out. Repeat on the opposite leg.

Quads

POSITION: Roll right over so the roller is on the tops of the fronts of your legs and lean to one side. Roll up and down and then switch to the other side.

Lats

POSITION: Lie on the roller so that it is under your armpit, and roll from your armpit to your hip along your lat with your bottom arm extended or bent behind your head.

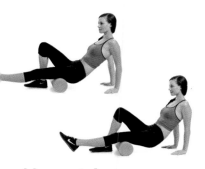

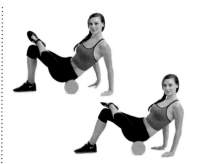

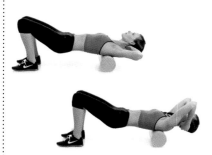

Hamstrings

POSITION: With your leg straight out and your hands behind you with your weight back on your arms, roll from the top of your leg where your hamstring goes into your hip right down to your knee. Put your weight on one leg and roll up and down, and then massage the other leg.

Hips

POSITION: Sit on the foam roller, cross your left leg over your right, and lean toward your left hip, putting your weight on your left hand. Roll on your glute and stop if you feel a spot that feels like a knot. Switch sides.

Thoracic Mobilization

POSITION: With the foam roller across your upper back, place your hands behind your head to support your neck. With your elbows up and out, roll slowly up and down your upper back as you extend and relax back onto the roller.

RAMP 2: Half-Kneeling Hip Flexor Stretch with Rotation and Rear Foot Elevated

This is described on page 000.

Hold for
30
seconds

REPEAT
on the
other
side

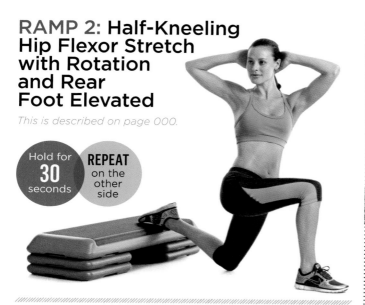

Perform
5
reps

REPEAT
on the
other
side

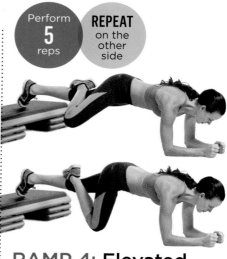

RAMP 4: Elevated Plank Hip External Rotation Knee Raise

This is an excellent exercise to wake up your core and the external rotators of the hip.

START: Get into the plank position from Phase One, but this time elevate your feet onto a small box or step, ideally putting your feet at the same height as your hips. Bend your right leg, touching your right foot to your left knee in a dancer's "passé" position, with the knee pointing toward the floor.

MOVEMENT: Keeping a stable plank position, rotate from your right hip, raising your right knee to the side while maintaining contact with the right foot and left knee, similar to the external hip rotation movement of the Side Lying Clam Shell you did in Phase One, or the Quadruped Hydrant in Phase Two. Lift the knee up, hold it in the top position for 1 second, and then lower back down and repeat. While you are doing this, be sure to keep your entire upper body and lower back completely still. Don't start to twist or get tension up in your neck and shoulders. Once you complete all of the reps on one side, switch sides.

RAMP 3: Hip/Thigh Extension

START: Lie on your back on the floor, bend your left leg at a 90-degree angle, and straighten your right leg. Your hands should be palms up and your arms 45 degrees away from your body. Lift your entire body up 1 inch by pushing off your left foot.

MOVEMENT: Continue to lift until your entire body is in a straight line and your thighs are parallel to each other. The only parts of your body that are in contact with the floor are your arms, upper back, and left foot. Lower to 1 inch off the floor, pause, and repeat for the prescribed number of repetitions. Be sure to keep your hips in a straight line. Repeat with the other side. The extended leg can be bent, weighted with an ankle weight, or tucked.

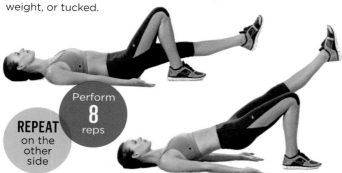

REPEAT
on the
other
side

Perform
8
reps

RAMP 5: Open Half-Kneeling with Thoracic Reach

START: Kneel on your left knee with your right foot flat on the floor and turned out from your body, forming a 90-degree angle with your left leg. Place your left hand just in front of your left leg and reach your right arm toward the ceiling.

MOVEMENT: Bring your right arm down and through your left arm and left leg and then reach back up toward the ceiling. Repeat.

Perform **5** reps

REPEAT on the other side

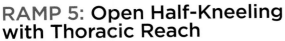
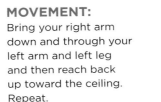
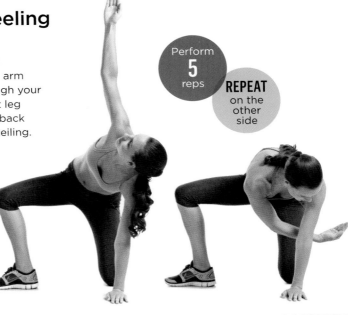

RAMP 6: Squat to Stand 2

START: You'll feel your entire body waking up doing this movement! Stand with feet slightly wider than shoulder-width apart, with your arms reaching overhead as high as you can.

MOVEMENT: Keeping both arms reaching overhead, bend over at your waist to touch your toes, keeping your legs straight and stretching out your hamstrings. Keeping your hands on your toes, drop your hips down into a squat position with your knees on the outside of your arms. Staying in a full squat position, reach both arms overhead, then stand up to return to the start position and repeat.

Perform **10** reps

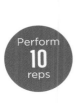
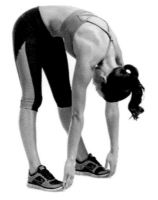
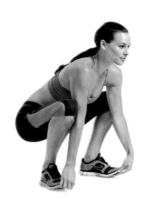
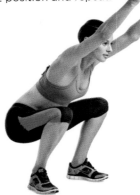

RAMP 7: Inchworm

START: Stand with your feet shoulder-width apart.

MOVEMENT: Bend at your hips and touch your hands to the floor as close to your feet as possible, feeling a stretch in your hamstrings. Walk your hands one at a time away from your feet and continue walking until you're in a pushup position. From there, continue walking your hands even farther, until you've walked out as far as you can while keeping your back flat. The goal is to eventually get your hands well past your head so you are completely stretched out. From here, walk your feet in toward your hands like an inchworm and repeat. Be sure to keep your feet pointing straight ahead for the entire set.

Perform
5
reps

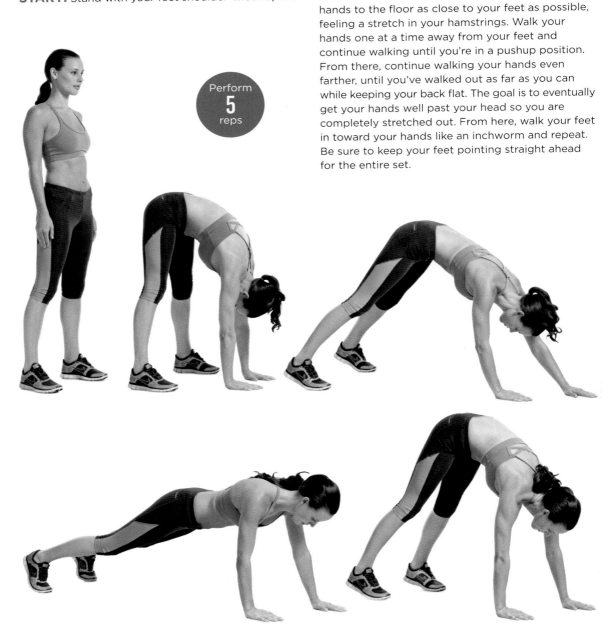

RAMP 8: Open Half-Kneeling with Ankle Mobilization

START: Kneel on your left knee with your right foot flat on the floor and turned out from your body, forming a 90-degree angle with your left leg. Your body should be upright with good posture and your hips under your shoulders.

MOVEMENT: Lunge to the right, driving your right knee over your right toe while keeping your heel down. You'll feel a stretch in your ankle and your inner thigh.

Perform
5
reps

REPEAT
on the
other
side

Perform
10
reps

REPEAT
on the
other
side

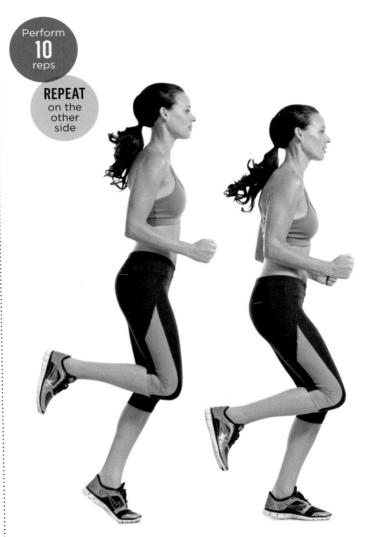

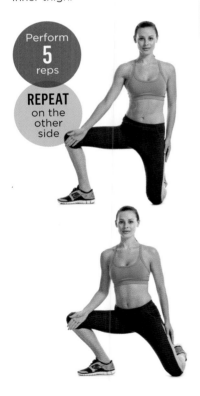

RAMP 9: Forward/Back Hop

START: Stand on your left leg.

MOVEMENT: Imagine there's a line drawn horizontally on the floor in front of you. Hop over the line with your left leg and land on your left foot. Then hop backward over the line to the start position. Keep the hops small and pretend the floor is hot. Perform 10 on your left leg and 10 on your right leg. Again, you're waking up your nervous system!

RAMP 10:
Forward/Back Leg Swing

START: Stand alongside a wall with your feet shoulder-width apart. Place one hand on the wall for support and place your other hand on your hip. Shift your weight to inside leg and lift the outside leg, starting to let it swing from front to back.

MOVEMENT: Keeping your upper body perfectly still, start to swing the leg a little higher to the front and a little higher to the back as you start to work the range of motion and get your hip loose and warmed up while also engaging your core and keeping it perfectly still. Complete your reps and then switch sides.

Perform
8
reps

REPEAT
on the
other
side

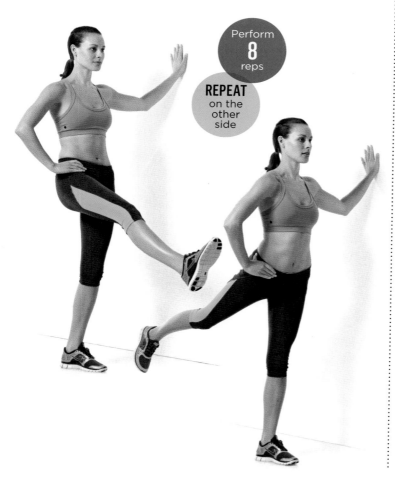

Perform
10
reps

REPEAT
on the
other
side

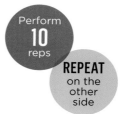

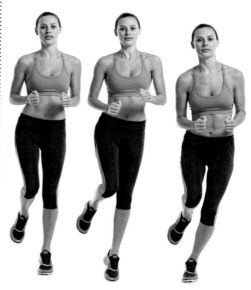

RAMP 11:
Lateral Hop

START: Stand on your left leg.

MOVEMENT: Imagine there's a line drawn on the floor to your left. Hop over the line with your left leg, land on your left foot, and then hop back over, still landing on the same foot. Keep the hops small and, again, pretend the floor is hot. Perform 10 on your left leg, then 10 on your right leg (starting with the imaginary line at your right side).

RAMP 12:
Cross-in-Front Lunge

START: Stand with your feet shoulder-width apart and your arms at your sides.

MOVEMENT: Cross your right foot over your left and step about 2 feet forward and to the left of your left foot. Bend both knees, in a movement very similar to a curtsy. Keep your hips facing forward. You should feel a stretch across your right hip as you lunge. Return to the start position and repeat on the other side.

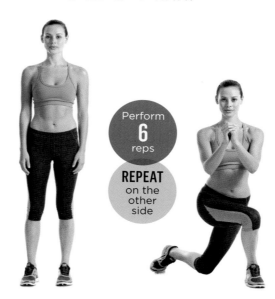

Perform
6
reps

REPEAT
on the other side

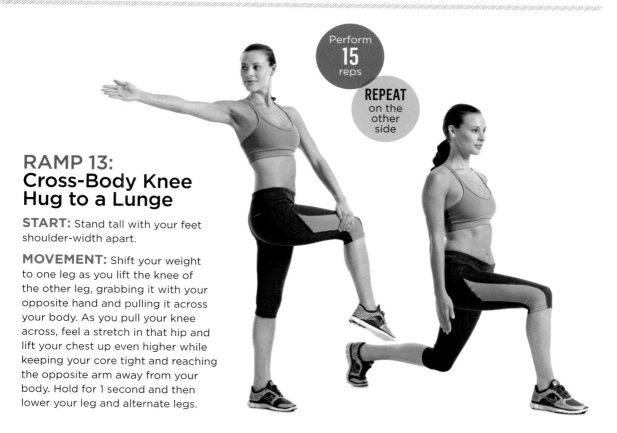

Perform
15
reps

REPEAT
on the other side

RAMP 13:
Cross-Body Knee Hug to a Lunge

START: Stand tall with your feet shoulder-width apart.

MOVEMENT: Shift your weight to one leg as you lift the knee of the other leg, grabbing it with your opposite hand and pulling it across your body. As you pull your knee across, feel a stretch in that hip and lift your chest up even higher while keeping your core tight and reaching the opposite arm away from your body. Hold for 1 second and then lower your leg and alternate legs.

PHASE 3: Strength
Workout 1

First do the Get Moving RAMP exercises. Then perform the following exercises as described in the chart.

Exercise	Sets	Reps	Speed	Rest
CORE				
1 Wood Chop	1-2	12 ea side	Mod	45 secs
POWER				
2 Box Jump/ Jump Squat	1-2	5-6	Fast	1 min
STRENGTH				
3A Deadlift	2-3	12	Mod	1 min
3B T-Pushup	2-3	6 ea side	Mod	None
3C Rear-Foot Elevated Split Squat	2-3	12 ea side	Mod	None
3D Open Half-Kneeling with Thoracic Reach	2-3	5 ea side	Slow	None
4A Single Arm Push Press	2-3	12 ea side	Slow	1 min
4B Single Leg Romanian Deadlift with Single Arm Row	2-3	12 ea side	Slow	None
4C Half-Kneeling Hip Flexor Stretch with Rotation and Rear Foot Elevated	2-3	30 secs ea side	Slow	None
FINISHER				
5 Jump Squat	2-4	20	On the minute	1 min

1 Wood Chop

Including a rotational movement as part of your workout is extremely important and often forgotten. The Wood Chop is an excellent full body exercise working the rotational movement.

START: Stand tall with your feet shoulder-width apart. If you have a band to use, hook it under one of your feet and grab the handles, or if you have a dumbbell, grasp the dumbbell with both hands. Both hands will be clasped and to the side of your leg.

MOVEMENT: Keeping your arms straight, pull the weight straight across your body at a diagonal. Keep your eyes on your hands as you do the movement. Return to the start position under control and repeat. Think about bending your legs from side to side, shifting your weight back and forth as you pull across your body, making this a whole-body exercise. Your shoulders and eyes should follow your hands as you twist, and your knees should be bent slightly.

Perform
12
reps

REPEAT
on the
other
side

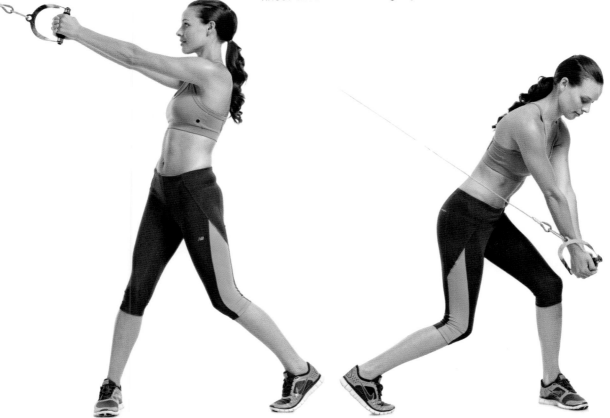

2 Box Jump/Jump Squat

This exercise is as much a mind-set exercise as it is a physical exercise. Start with a small box that you know you can land on top of and remember the words, "I can jump on this box." As soon as you doubt yourself, you'll be less likely to land on the box.

START: Stand in front of a sturdy step or box that can hold your body weight.

MOVEMENT: Bend both knees and jump, landing on the box with both feet at the same time with a soft landing (think "catlike"). As you land, your knees should not buckle in but should instead stay tracking over your toes while you support your landing by engaging your glutes and core. Step back down off the box one foot at a time; do not jump off the box. Repeat. If you don't have a box to jump on to, then perform Jump Squats.

Perform
5-6
reps

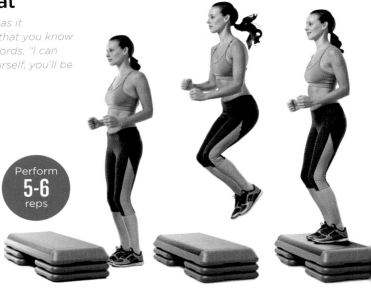

3A Deadlift

START: Place dumbbells, kettlebells, or a barbell on the floor right in front of your toes. Bend your knees so that your thighs are slightly above parallel to the floor, but keep your shoulders directly over your hands in front of you. Keep your head in neutral alignment and grab the dumbbells, kettlebells, or barbell.

MOVEMENT: Keeping a normal arch in your lower back, stand straight up and bring your hips forward. At the top you should be standing straight up with your chest tall, legs straight, and your arms in front of your thighs. Think about pushing the earth away from you, like a jumping action rather than a lifting action. Lower under control to the floor (by flexing your hips and then your knees) to complete the repetition.

Perform
12
reps

> **OPTION:** *If you are unable to maintain a neutral spine with full range of motion, set the weights on a small box or step instead of trying to reach for the floor.*

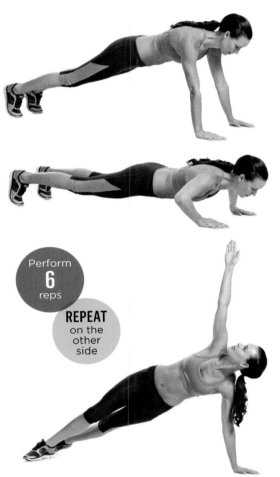

3C Rear-Foot Elevated Split Squat

Perform as described on page 140. Last phase, you performed this exercise with your foot on a stable surface. You can repeat that again or place your foot in a TRX strap, creating instability and making you work even harder. You got this!

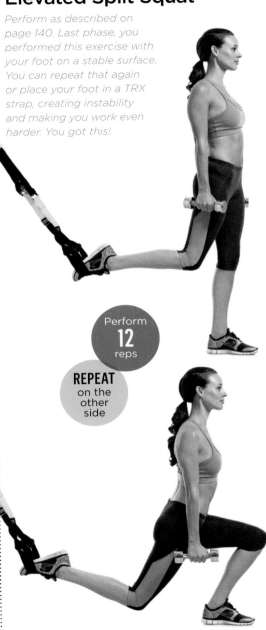

Perform
6
reps

REPEAT
on the
other
side

Perform
12
reps

REPEAT
on the
other
side

3B T-Pushup

START: Assume a standard pushup position.

MOVEMENT: Perform a pushup, then transfer all your weight to one hand as you rotate your body to reach up and behind you with the opposite hand. Keep both feet on the floor while pivoting to turn. Your arms should be in a straight line so that your body forms a T shape. Alternate sides. Once this becomes easy, lift both your arm and the foot on the same side off the floor after each pushup, so you make an X shape with your arms and legs. Holding hexagon-shaped dumbbells in your hands can also increase the intensity, or wear a weight vest.

3D Open Half-Kneeling with Thoracic Reach

START: Kneel on your left knee with your right foot flat on the floor and turned out from your body, forming a 90-degree angle with your left leg. Place your left hand just in front of your left leg and reach your right arm toward the ceiling.

MOVEMENT: Bring your right arm down and through your left arm and left leg and then reach back up toward the ceiling. Repeat. Then switch sides.

Perform
5
reps

REPEAT
on the
other
side

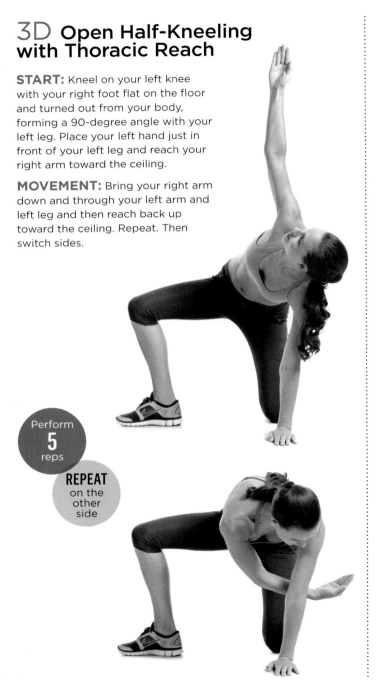

Perform
12
reps

REPEAT
on the
other
side

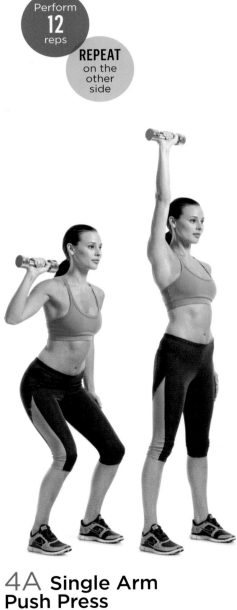

4A Single Arm Push Press

Perform as described on page 133.

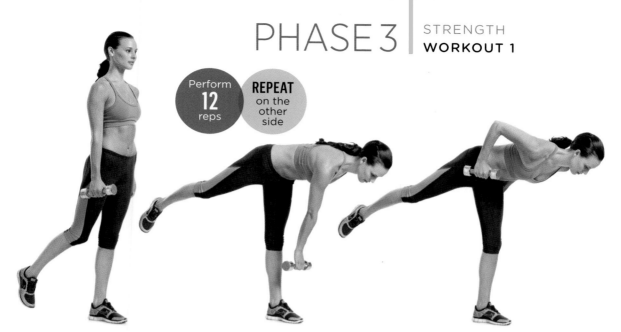

Perform **12** reps   **REPEAT** on the other side

4B Single Leg Romanian Deadlift with Single Arm Row

Perform as described on page 135, but as you are coming back up, stop when your back is neutral and the weight is hanging straight down and row the weight up. Lower the weight and then stand up. Repeat. Switch sides.

4C
Half-Kneeling Hip Flexor Stretch with Rotation and Rear Foot Elevated

Perform as described on page 56.

Hold for **30** seconds

REPEAT on the other side

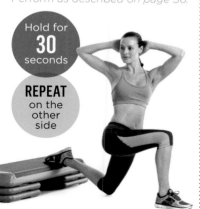

5 Jump Squat

Perform a Body Weight Speed Squat as described on page 202, except from the bottom of the squat generate enough power to jump off the floor into the air. As you land, return to the squat position and repeat.

Perform **20** reps in a minute

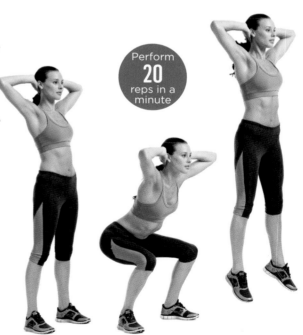

PHASE 3: Strength
Workout 2

First do the Get Moving RAMP exercises. Then perform the following exercises as described in the chart.

Exercise	Sets	Reps	Speed	Rest
CORE				
1 **Body Saw**	1-2	8	Mod	45 secs
POWER				
2 **Jump Lunge**	1-2	8 ea side	Fast	1 min
STRENGTH				
3A **Front Squat with Dumbbells or Barbell**	2-3	12	Mod	1 min
3B **Chinup with Band**	2-3	12	Slow	None
3C **Cross-Over Stepup**	2-3	12 ea side	Mod	None
3D **Open Half-Kneeling with Ankle Mobilization**	2-3	5 ea side	Slow	None
4A **Two-Point Dumbbell Row**	2-3	12 ea side	Slow	None
4B **Lateral Lunge with Contra Load and Overhead Press**	2-3	12 ea side	Mod	None
4C **Hip/Thigh Extension**	2-3	12 ea side	Mod	None
FINISHER				
5 **Single Arm Swing**	2-4	20 (10 ea side)	On the minute	Rest until min is up

1 Body Saw

START: Place your feet in the TRX and get on your elbows in a plank position.

MOVEMENT: Start with a very small movement pushing your body back toward the TRX by opening up the angle under your arm and putting an increased demand on your core. Return to the start position and repeat. Each time you do this exercise, you can try to get a little more range.

OPTION: *You can also do this exercise with your body weight, with your feet on the ground.*

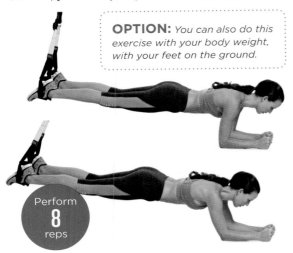

Perform
8
reps

2 Jump Lunge

START: Stand at the top of a lunge with your feet split apart.

MOVEMENT: Lower yourself to the bottom of a lunge and then explosively launch yourself into the air, exchanging your legs in midair. Upon landing (your feet will be opposite of where they were at the start), go into another lunge and repeat for the required time period.

Perform
8
reps

REPEAT
on the other side

OPTION: *Hold on to a TRX while performing this exercise to make it easier.*

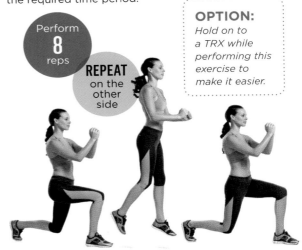

3A Front Squat with Dumbbells or Barbell

START: Stand with your feet slightly wider than shoulder-width apart and either hold dumbbells at shoulder height or hold a barbell on your back (use a squat rack to safely load the bar). Your chest should be up, hips underneath your shoulders, and core engaged.

MOVEMENT: Bending at your knees and hips and pushing your knees out, lower into a full squat position, keeping your torso as upright as possible. Try to get your hips below parallel so that you can achieve maximum range of motion. Use your legs and hips to drive yourself back up to the start position and repeat.

Perform
12
reps

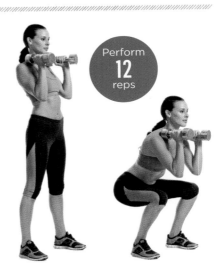

3B Chinup with Band

Women can do chinups—we just need to work at them! They are a great example of how much strength you have compared to your weight.

START: If you're a beginner, 6 to 8 unassisted chinups might not be doable—yet. So you can use a band for assistance, or do Negative Chinups. As you get stronger, use a thinner and thinner band until you're doing chinups without the band. To use a band for assistance, hang from a chinup bar with a band looped around the bar and around one knee. Your hands should be facing you and fully extended. To perform Negative Chinups: You'll need a step high enough to give you a boost up to the top of the chinup, where you'll start the exercise. Very slowly, lower yourself down, going as slowly and as controlled as possible.

MOVEMENT: Pull yourself up to the bar until your chin is over the bar and then return to the start position. Think about bringing your elbows to your sides, which will ensure that you're using your back to pull yourself up. The band should act as support to help lift you up. The thicker the band, the easier it will be for you to pull your body weight up. Don't swing your legs or kick to cheat your way up. As you get stronger, eventually ditch the band and do chinups on your own.

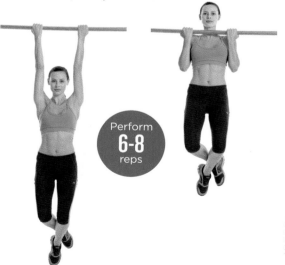

Perform
6-8
reps

3C Cross-Over Stepup

This move takes the stepup and turns you sideways, switching on your outer thighs more and working in a different plane of motion. You'll really feel this in your butt!

START: Holding a dumbbell in each hand, stand alongside a bench or step that can support your body weight. Place your outside foot flat on the step, crossing over your body while keeping your hips square, sideways to the step.

MOVEMENT: Shift your weight onto the foot on the step, driving yourself up onto the step and balancing on the working leg. Slowly lower yourself back down to the start position and repeat. Then switch sides.

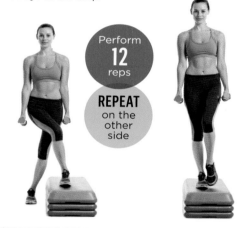

Perform
12
reps

REPEAT
on the
other
side

3D Open Half-Kneeling with Ankle Mobilization

Perform this exercise as described on page 197.

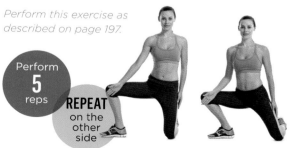

Perform
5
reps

REPEAT
on the
other
side

4A Two-Point Dumbbell Row

This is a progression from the Three-Point Dumbbell Row you did in Phase One.

START: Bend over at your hips, holding one dumbbell straight down. Your back should be flat and your spine in a straight line.

MOVEMENT: Row the dumbbell up to your side by squeezing your shoulder blades back and together. Then return to the start position and repeat.

Perform
12
reps

REPEAT
on the other side

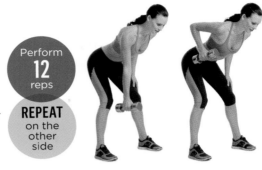

4B Lateral Lunge with Contra Load and Overhead Press

Perform as described on page 66, except as you finish the lateral lunge and bring your feet together, bring the dumbbell up to shoulder height and press it overhead. Repeat on the same side for the prescribed number of reps. Switch sides.

Perform
12
reps

REPEAT
on the other side

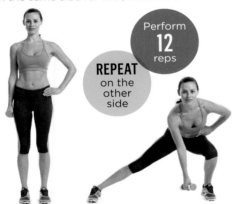
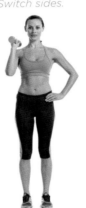
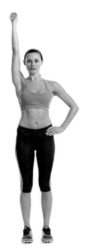

4C Hip/Thigh Extension

Perform this exercise as described on page 194.

Perform
12
reps

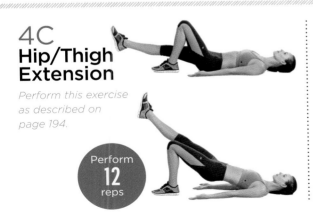

5 Single Arm Swing

Perform this exercise as described on page 77.

Perform
20
reps

(10 on each side) on the minute

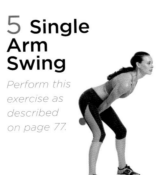
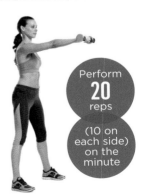

PHASE 3: Countdown
Metabolic Workout

Start with 10 reps of each exercise and only do evens this phase—after 10 reps, do 8 reps, then 6, 4, 2. Next time you perform the Countdown Metabolic Workout, add one tier, doing 12, 10, 8, 6, 4, 2. The third time you'll perform 14, 12, 10, 8, 6, 4, 2.

Sprint or jump rope for 40 seconds one time at the end of each round. Rest for 2 minutes and repeat for 8 reps, 6 reps, etc.

Exercise	Sets	Reps	Speed	Rest
CIRCUIT				
1A Jump Squat	5	10*	Fast	None
1B Deadlift with High Pull	5	10*	Fast	None
1C Super Plank	5	10*	Fast	None
1D Alternating Dumbbell or Kettlebell Clean	5	10*	Fast	None
1E Alternating Reverse Lunge with Overhead Reach	5	10 ea side*	Fast	None
CARDIO				
Jump Rope		40 secs after each round		
REST				
Active Recovery		Rest for 2 min		

* Perform 10 reps of each (in set 1), 8 reps of each (in set 2), 6 reps of each (in set 3), 4 reps of each (in set 4), 2 reps of each (in set 5)

1A Jump Squat

Perform a Body Weight Speed Squat as described on page 67, except from the bottom of the squat generate enough power to jump off the floor into the air. As you land, return to the squat position and repeat.

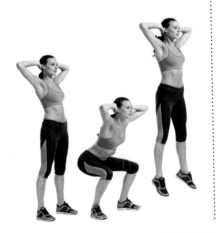

1B Deadlift with High Pull

Perform a Deadlift with lighter dumbbells or a bar (see page 77), but as you lift the weight, generate enough power to "High Pull" the weight (see page 64). Return to the start position and repeat.

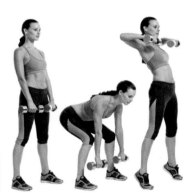

1C Super Plank

START: Get into a plank position with your elbows directly under your shoulders and your head, upper back, hips, and ankles all in one straight line.

MOVEMENT: Walk up onto one hand and then the other hand so you are in a pushup position. Then lower back to the start position by placing one elbow down and then the other. Alternate the arm you go up on first and lower to first.

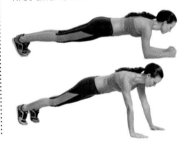

1D Alternating Dumbbell or Kettlebell Clean

Perform the Kettlebell Clean as described on page 79. This exercise can be performed with a kettlebell or dumbbell.

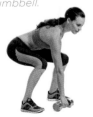
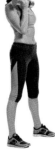

1E Alternating Reverse Lunge with Overhead Reach

START: Stand with your feet shoulder-width apart.

MOVEMENT: Step back into a lunge while reaching both arms overhead. Drive off your front leg and return to the start position while lowering your arms. Repeat on the other side. Feel free to hold on to a medicine ball or dumbbell to increase the difficulty.

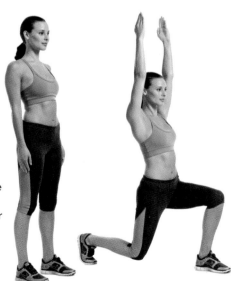

PHASE 3: Complex
Metabolic Workout

First do the Get Moving RAMP exercises. Then perform 8 of each of the following exercises one after the other, moving as fast as possible. Rest for 90 seconds and then repeat. Perform the circuit four times.

Exercise	Sets	Reps	Speed	Rest
CIRCUIT				
1A Left Arm Dumbbell Deadlift	1*	8	Fast	None
1B Left Arm Dumbbell Clean	1	8	Fast	None
1C Left Arm Offset Dumbbell Goblet Squat	1	8	Fast	None
1D Left Arm Push Press	1	8	Fast	None
2A Right Arm Dumbbell Deadlift	1	8	Fast	None
2B Right Arm Dumbbell Clean	1	8	Fast	None
2C Right Arm Offset Dumbbell Goblet Squat	1	8	Fast	None
2D Right Arm Push Press	1	8	Fast	None
REST				
Active Recovery	Rest for 90 secs			

* Perform 4 rounds of the circuit, resting 90 seconds after each.

1A
Left Arm Dumbbell Deadlift

Perform as described on page 141.

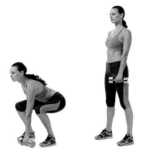

1B
Left Arm Dumbbell Clean

Perform as described on page 211.

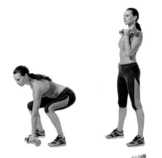

1C
Left Arm Offset Dumbbell Goblet Squat

Perform as described on page 134.

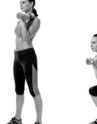
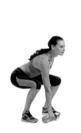

1D
Left Arm Push Press

Perform as described on page 204.

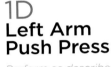
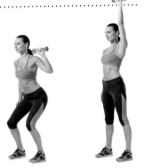
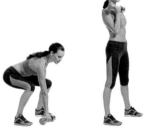

2A
Right Arm Dumbbell Deadlift

Perform as described on page 141.

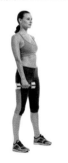

2B
Right Arm Dumbbell Clean

Perform as described on page 211.

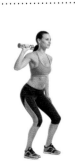

2C
Right Arm Offset Dumbbell Goblet Squat

Perform as described on page 134.

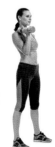
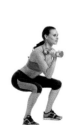

2D
Right Arm Push Press

Perform as described on page 204.

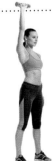

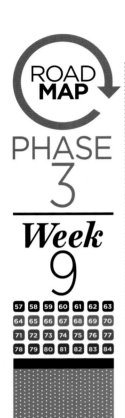

ROAD MAP

PHASE 3

Week **9**

57	58	59	60	61	62	63
64	65	66	67	68	69	70
71	72	73	74	75	76	77
78	79	80	81	82	83	84

It's Week Nine, the final phase!

As you head into Phase Three, it might be tempting to relax at this point and allow yourself to slip back into old habits—maybe Lazy Cheats or skipping workouts. Don't do it! You've worked too hard to sabotage your progress. It's more important than ever to be vigilant about sticking to your mission statement and remind yourself of your goals.

Each time you overcome taking the "comfortable" way out (sleeping in, taking the elevator), you are continually retraining your mind and body—and you're becoming a new person with new habits. Recommit to the plan and to yourself over the next 4 weeks. Make every choice a positive one!

Week Nine
Plan of Attack:

Get your journal out and take inventory of your splurges so far.

Remember, the best way to keep track of your food intake is to write it down! Please don't rely on your memory. At this point you should have had no more than 24 splurges in the last 8 weeks. If you have had more than that, it may creep up on you at your next Jeans Check. But all is not lost.

Commit this last month to really stepping it up and use only one splurge a week. You can still make a lot of progress over the last 4 weeks. Stay focused.

Week Nine Grocery List

PRODUCE

- Apples
- Bananas
- Berries
- Lemons
- Asparagus
- Avocado (1)
- Bell peppers
- Cabbage
- Carrots
- Celery
- Cucumber
- Greens, mixed
- Portobello mushroom (1)
- Spinach, baby
- Tomatoes
- Basil
- Cilantro (optional)
- Garlic

DAIRY & EGGS

- Cheese, shredded mozzarella
- Eggs
- Goat cheese
- Greek yogurt, 2% (plain)
- Milk, 2% (cow, soy, or almond)

BAKERY

- Corn tortillas
- Ezekiel bread
- Ezekiel English muffin
- Ezekiel tortillas

MEAT, DELI & SEAFOOD

- Chicken breasts, boneless, skinless (2 pounds)
- Mahi mahi (or tilapia)
- Shrimp
- Tilapia
- Turkey breast, ground

GROCERY & PANTRY

- Almonds, raw
- Beans, black, canned (15 ounces)
- Broth, chicken or vegetable
- Chickpeas
- Fruit, dried
- Muir Glen Organic Marinara Sauce
- Oatmeal (rolled oats)
- Olives
- Peanut butter, natural
- Salsa
- Whey protein powder

FROZEN

- Berries

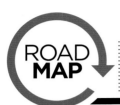

PHASE 3

Week 9

57	58	59	60	61	62	63
64	65	66	67	68	69	70
71	72	73	74	75	76	77
78	79	80	81	82	83	84

Day 57

TODAY'S FOCUS ✓

ACTION: Give 100 percent.
Today you start the third and final phase of the program. The third phase progresses even further from the last phase, so you may find it more challenging—but there's nothing you can't handle! Tackle your workout today with everything you have as you learn the new exercises. You have built a base strength at this point and are ready to take your training up a notch. Give it 100 percent effort.

WORKOUT

PHASE 3: STRENGTH 1

MENU PLAN 🍴

Take supplements: 1 to 2 grams omega-3s, multivitamin, and 1,000 IU vitamin D
Plus 1 serving of Greens+

Breakfast
Ezekiel French Toast (see opposite)
1 cup fresh fruit

Snack
1 cup 2% Greek yogurt topped with 2 tablespoons chopped raw almonds

Lunch
Grilled Chicken Salad (page 104) and 2 tablespoons Homemade Vinaigrette (page 151)

Snack
Post-Workout Shake (page 85)

Dinner
4-ounce turkey burger on portobello mushroom
Side Salad (page 83)

Day 58

TODAY'S FOCUS

ACTION: Tune in to your feel-good moments.

By this point, you probably have a moment every once in a while where you catch a glimpse of yourself in the mirror or you notice new definition on your body. Or, you rock one of your workouts and you think, "I feel strong and sexy! I rock!" Remember them when you are tempted to give in to a Lazy Cheat or skip a workout. Close your eyes and remember how great you felt at that moment and how every ounce of effort is totally worth it.

WORKOUT

DAY OFF: Active Recovery, optional 20-minute interval workout, or repeat this week's metabolic workout.

MENU PLAN

Take supplements: 1 to 2 grams omega-3s, multivitamin, and 1,000 IU vitamin D
Plus 1 serving of Greens+

Breakfast
*1 cup cooked oatmeal
  (made with 1 cup 2% milk)*
¼ cup dried fruit

Snack
1 apple
1 tablespoon natural peanut butter

Lunch
4 ounces grilled chicken breast
*1 slice Ezekiel bread topped with 1 ounce
  goat cheese and sliced tomato*

Snack
Post-Workout Shake (page 85)

Dinner
5 ounces cooked tilapia
*1 cup steamed chopped asparagus,
  roasted with 2 teaspoons olive oil*

Ezekiel French Toast

*1 egg
¼ cup 2% almond,
  soy, or cow milk
¼ teaspoon ground
  cinnamon
1 slice Ezekiel bread*

In a medium bowl, combine the egg, milk, and cinnamon; whisk well. Heat a nonstick skillet over medium heat and spray with cooking spray. Dip the bread in the egg mixture and coat well on both sides. Transfer the bread to the hot skillet and cook for 2 to 3 minutes per side, or until golden brown. Serve topped with fresh fruit. Makes 1 serving.

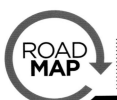

PHASE 3

Week 9

57 58 59 60 61 62 63
64 65 66 67 68 69 70
71 72 73 74 75 76 77
78 79 80 81 82 83 84

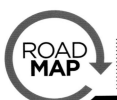

Day 59

TODAY'S FOCUS

ACTION: Check your portions.

I don't want you to worry about counting calories or grams. These take care of themselves if you eat the right amount of the right foods, 90 percent of the time. This challenge is about taking the focus off of the numbers—no scales, no calories, no points, no grams— no obsessing! When it comes to portions, throughout the day you should eat a portion of protein and two portions of fruits or vegetables at each meal A portion of protein should be about the size and width of the palm of your hand, and a portion of vegetables and fruits should be at least the size of your fist.

WORKOUT

PHASE 3: STRENGTH 2

MENU PLAN

Take supplements: 1 to 2 grams omega-3s, multivitamin, and 1,000 IU vitamin D
Plus 1 serving of Greens+

Breakfast
Ezekiel French Toast (page 217)
1 cup fresh fruit

Snack
1 cup 2% Greek yogurt
½ cup fresh berries

Lunch
Fish Tacos: *5 ounces cooked mahi mahi or tilapia, shredded cabbage, and salsa in 2 corn tortillas*

Snack
Post-Workout Shake (page 85)

Dinner
Grilled Chicken Salad (page 104) and 2 tablespoons Homemade Vinaigrette (page 151)

Day 60

TODAY'S FOCUS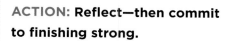

ACTION: Reflect—then commit to finishing strong.

Congratulations! Today marks the 60th day of your journey. We talked about how the first 30 days set you up to succeed. Now, after 60 days, you have doubled your chances of success by truly changing your habits and your lifestyle. Way to go! Reflect on your successes and what you have learned from the challenges you've faced over the past 60 days, then get focused and commit to finishing strong.

WORKOUT

DAY OFF: Active Recovery or complete day of rest.

MENU PLAN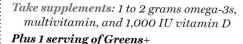

Take supplements: 1 to 2 grams omega-3s, multivitamin, and 1,000 IU vitamin D
Plus 1 serving of Greens+

Breakfast
1 cup cooked oatmeal
(made with 1 cup 2% milk)
¼ cup berries

Snack
1 cup 2% Greek yogurt
1 cup fresh berries

Lunch
Chopped Salad with Shrimp (page 161)

Snack
Post-Workout Shake (page 85)

Dinner
5 ounces grilled chicken breast topped with a thin layer of Pesto (page 175)
1 cup sliced cucumber

Do I Need a Food Scale?

I do think occasionally measuring and weighing foods with a scale is helpful because it helps you readjust your eyes. The problem? It's not realistic to carry around a scale with you all the time. Here's a better tool: your hand.

- **1 cup = your fist**
- **1 table-spoon = your thumb (from base to tip)**
- **1 teaspoon = your thumb tip (from knuckle to tip)**
- **3 ounces = the thick-ness and size of the palm of your hand (excluding fingers)**

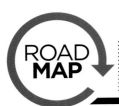

ROAD MAP

Day 61

PHASE 3

Week 9

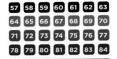

57	58	59	60	61	62	63
64	65	66	67	68	69	70
71	72	73	74	75	76	77
78	79	80	81	82	83	84

TODAY'S FOCUS ✓

ACTION: Plan your splurges.

Admit it: How many Lazy Cheats have you used? Are you enjoying your splurges or are you wasting them? You'll start to feel deprived if you waste them on food you didn't really want. The secret is to stick to the plan 100 percent for each meal—except three splurge meals each week. For those three meals, pick times and places when you can really enjoy the experience and the food. The great part is that if you do it right, you can actually have your cake and look great too!

WORKOUT

PHASE 3: STRENGTH 1

MENU PLAN

Take supplements: 1 to 2 grams omega-3s, multivitamin, and 1,000 IU vitamin D
Plus 1 serving of Greens+

Breakfast
Breakfast Wrap (page 112)
1 banana

Snack
1 apple
1 tablespoon natural peanut butter

Lunch
Avocado and Chickpea Salad (page 118)

Snack
Post-Workout Shake (page 85)

Dinner
Chicken Parmesan (page 171)
Side Salad (page 83) and 1 tablespoon Homemade Vinaigrette (page 151)

Day 62

TODAY'S FOCUS

ACTION: Treat yourself today!
You are three-quarters of the way through and you deserve a reward. Treat yourself today. Buy yourself a new workout outfit, get a massage, book a pedicure, or do all three!

WORKOUT

PHASE 3: COUNTDOWN METABOLIC

MENU PLAN

Take supplements: 1 to 2 grams omega-3s, multivitamin, and 1,000 IU vitamin D
Plus 1 serving of Greens+

Breakfast
1 cup cooked oatmeal (made with 1 cup 2% milk)
¼ cup dried fruit

Snack
1 hard-cooked egg
Cucumber slices

Lunch
4 ounces grilled chicken breast
1 slice Ezekiel bread topped with 1 ounce goat cheese and sliced tomato

Snack
Post-Workout Shake (page 85)

Dinner
1 serving Black Bean Soup (page 97). Refrigerate the second serving for dinner on Day 63.

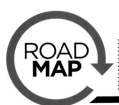

PHASE 3

Week 9

57	58	59	60	61	62	63
64	65	66	67	68	69	70
71	72	73	74	75	76	77
78	79	80	81	82	83	84

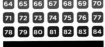

Day 63

TODAY'S FOCUS ✓

ACTION: Make some swaps.
Today is your planning day, which should be part of your weekly ritual by now. Plan ahead for the next 24 hours and even through the next week. Over these final 3 weeks, try to increase your fish intake, swapping out red meat for salmon, or turkey for white fish. Fish is the best source of protein, and the omega-3s it contains make it the best "bang for your buck" when it comes to a protein source.

WORKOUT 🏃

DAY OFF: Active Recovery
or complete day of rest.

MENU PLAN 🍴

Take supplements: 1 to 2 grams omega-3s, multivitamin, and 1,000 IU vitamin D
Plus 1 serving of Greens+

Breakfast
Breakfast Wrap (page 112)

Snack
1 cup 2% Greek yogurt
1 cup fresh berries

Lunch
Ezekiel English Muffin Pizza: *1 Ezekiel English muffin topped with marinara sauce, vegetables (as desired), and ⅓ cup shredded mozzarella cheese**

*Bake at 400°F until cheese is melted.

Snack
Post-Workout Shake (page 85)

Dinner
1 serving Black Bean Soup (page 97; see Day 62)
Side Salad (page 83) and 1 tablespoon Homemade Vinaigrette (page 151)

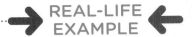
Change at Last

MARIA PALMA > dropped two sizes in 12 weeks

I was very skeptical that I could change my body. I walk 2 to 4 miles a day, ride my bike, or do P90X at home—but for the most part my body just stayed the same no matter how I ate or exercised. I have had type 1 diabetes for 26 years and being on insulin makes it hard to lose any weight. I just figured I was stuck with my body! When I started this program I had a muffin top, a belly, and arms that were starting to get flabby and did not look toned. This time I was determined not to give up.

The first 2 weeks my blood sugars were all over the place, and I was using muscles that obviously had not been used in a long time. But I kept doing the workouts every day and figuring out how to eat better. My family eats out a lot, mostly because I could never figure out what to make. Drop Two Sizes forced me to find healthy dinner recipes that even my 16-year-old son will eat. I'm happy to say we now eat at home most of the week and have found new family dinner favorites!

A real eye opener for me was when I tried on my jeans for the first time. I was shocked at how well they fit. The scale remained the same, but my butt now fit into these jeans! In 12 weeks I was able to trim my hips, lose most of my muffin top, flatten my stomach, and start to show some definition in my arms. I learned a lot and this experience will stay with me always.

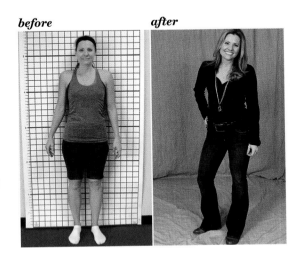

before   *after*

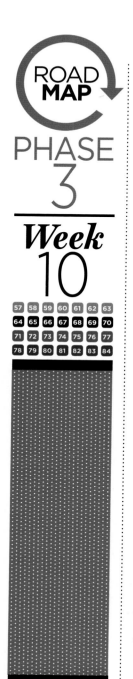

ROAD MAP

PHASE 3

Week 10

57	58	59	60	61	62	63
64	65	66	67	68	69	70
71	72	73	74	75	76	77
78	79	80	81	82	83	84

Welcome to Week Ten!

The finish line is close. You have only 3 weeks to go until you'll be strutting your stuff and looking fabulous wearing clothes at least two sizes smaller than when you started. It's time to step up your momentum as you're about to "peak." This is how athletes train—they train for events when they need to be at their peak performance, which keeps them constantly improving and working toward something. I believe the same is important for you. Over the next 3 weeks, think of your preparation as if you're running a marathon or competing in an event. Push yourself to succeed as though you will cross that finish line to the loudest roar of applause—because that's how it will feel to slide on your jeans or go shopping for new clothes with your best body ever.

Week Ten Plan of Attack:

You're about to embark on your last Jeans Check before the final try-on. If they are already fitting well, you can keep on cruising at the same speed.

If they are not quite there yet, it's time to put the pedal to the metal and ask yourself: What one thing do I need to change this week to have the biggest impact? Commit to making real changes to reach your goal.

Week Ten Grocery List

PRODUCE

- Berries (including strawberries)
- Lemons
- Limes
- Oranges
- Bell peppers
- Celery
- Cucumber
- Edamame, shelled (fresh or frozen)
- Greens, mixed
- Onion, red
- Onion, yellow
- Spinach, baby
- Tomatoes
- Basil
- Cilantro
- Parsley
- Tofu, extra-firm (5 ounces)

DAIRY & EGGS

- Cheese, feta (crumbled)
- Cheese, fresh mozzarella
- Cheese, Laughing Cow light
- Cheese, Parmesan
- Eggs
- Greek yogurt, 2% (plain)
- Milk, 2% (cow, soy, or almond)

BAKERY

- Ezekiel English muffins
- Ezekiel tortillas

MEAT, DELI & SEAFOOD

- Chicken breasts, boneless, skinless (1¼ pounds)
- Salmon, wild-caught (1 pound skinless)
- Shrimp
- Tilapia
- Turkey breast, ground

GROCERY & PANTRY

- Almond butter
- Almonds, raw
- Beans, black (canned)
- Beans, pinto, canned (15 ounces)
- Beans, red kidney, canned (15 ounces)
- Beer, dark
- Bread crumbs, dried
- Broth, low-sodium chicken
- Cumin, ground
- Quinoa
- Tomatoes, crushed (3 cans, 28 ounces each)
- Tuna, canned (water-packed)
- Whey protein powder

FROZEN

- Berries

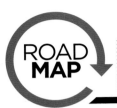

Day 64

PHASE 3
Week 10

57	58	59	60	61	62	63
64	65	66	67	68	69	70
71	72	73	74	75	76	77
78	79	80	81	82	83	84

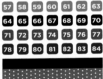

TODAY'S FOCUS ✓

Checkpoint: **Jeans Check**

Go ahead and get dressed! You might be surprised at how good it feels. The majority of our clients drop two sizes after 8 weeks—but some need the extra time to reach their goal. Wherever you are at this point, stay focused and complete the next 3 weeks strong to "peak" for the final week.

WORKOUT

PHASE 3: STRENGTH 2

MENU PLAN 🍴

Take supplements: 1 to 2 grams omega-3s, multivitamin, and 1,000 IU vitamin D
Plus 1 serving of Greens+

Breakfast
1 Ezekiel English muffin
1 tablespoon almond butter

Snack
2 pieces Laughing Cow light cheese
5 strawberries

Lunch
Asian Chicken Salad (page 94)
*   with Sesame Dressing (page 95)*

Snack
Post-Workout Shake (page 85)

Dinner
1 Salmon Burger (see opposite). You will use a second Salmon Burger for lunch on Day 65.
Side Salad (page 83) and 1 tablespoon Homemade Vinaigrette (page 151)

Day 65

TODAY'S FOCUS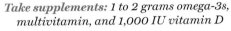

ACTION: A few tweaks to catapult your progress.

If your jeans didn't fit as well as you hoped yesterday, it's time to cut the cheese—literally. Eliminating cheese from your diet will cut down on extra sodium and calories that make a difference in your overall calorie intake and body composition. You'll still see some cheese in the upcoming menus, but it will be reduced. Swap cheese for another protein source such as hard-cooked eggs, nuts or seeds, or tuna to catapult your progress.

WORKOUT

DAY OFF: Active Recovery, optional 20-minute interval workout, or repeat this week's metabolic workout.

MENU PLAN

Take supplements: 1 to 2 grams omega-3s, multivitamin, and 1,000 IU vitamin D
Plus 1 serving of Greens+

Breakfast
Omelet Cup (page 181)
1 cup berries

Snack
A handful of raw almonds

Lunch
1 Salmon Burger (see Day 64)
3 cups mixed greens topped with lemon juice

Snack
Post-Workout Shake (page 85)

Dinner
1 serving Turkey Chili (page 181)

Salmon Burgers*

1 pound skinless wild-caught salmon, finely chopped
1 egg, beaten
¼ cup dried bread crumbs
¼ cup chopped onion
¼ cup chopped bell pepper
¼ teaspoon kosher salt
¼ cup finely chopped fresh herbs (such as basil, parsley, or cilantro)

In a large bowl, combine the salmon, egg, bread crumbs, onion, bell pepper, salt, and herbs. Form into 4 burgers. Grill or cook in a nonstick skillet for 8 to 10 minutes per side, or until cooked through. Makes 4.

*Refrigerate 1 burger for lunch on Day 65, and freeze the remaining 2.

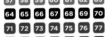

ROAD MAP

PHASE 3

Week 10

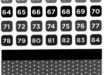

57	58	59	60	61	62	63
64	65	66	67	68	69	70
71	72	73	74	75	76	77
78	79	80	81	82	83	84

Day 66

TODAY'S FOCUS ✓

Checkpoint: **Water Check**
These last 3 weeks it is crucial that you are getting enough water. What is your strategy to know if you are getting enough water? Make this a priority.

WORKOUT 🏃

PHASE 3: STRENGTH 1

MENU PLAN 🍴

Take supplements: 1 to 2 grams omega-3s, multivitamin, and 1,000 IU vitamin D
Plus 1 serving of Greens+

Breakfast
1 cup 2% Greek yogurt
½ cup fresh berries
2 tablespoons chopped raw almonds

Snack
1 hard-cooked egg
5 strawberries

Lunch
Chicken Salad Wrap* (page 171)

*Make a double batch of the chicken salad mixture for lunch on Day 69.

Snack
Post-Workout Shake (page 85)

Dinner
4 ounces cooked shrimp, 1 cup diced tomatoes, and fresh basil
Side Salad (page 83) and 1 tablespoon Homemade Vinaigrette (page 151)

Day 67

TODAY'S FOCUS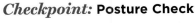

Checkpoint: **Posture Check**

How's your posture? It should reflect the growing confidence that comes with a more toned, fit physique. Keep your core engaged and your shoulders pulled down and back.

WORKOUT

DAY OFF: Active Recovery or complete day of rest.

MENU PLAN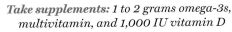

Take supplements: 1 to 2 grams omega-3s, multivitamin, and 1,000 IU vitamin D
Plus 1 serving of Greens+

Breakfast
1 Ezekiel English muffin
1 tablespoon almond butter

Snack
1 hard-cooked egg
Cucumber slices

Lunch
Quinoa Salad*: *¾ cup cooked quinoa, ½ cup diced cucumber, ½ cup diced bell pepper, ¼ cup black beans, 2 tablespoons crumbled feta cheese, 2 teaspoons olive oil, and freshly squeezed lime juice*
3 ounces diced cooked chicken breast, canned (water-packed) tuna, or cooked fish

*Make a double batch for lunch on Day 68.

Snack
Post-Workout Shake (page 85)

Dinner
5 ounces cooked chicken breast
Cucumber Salad: *1 cup sliced cucumber topped with thinly sliced red onion, 2 teaspoons extra virgin olive oil, and salt, pepper, and rice vinegar to taste*

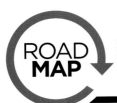

ROAD MAP

Day 68

PHASE
3

Week
10

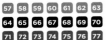
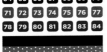

57 58 59 60 61 62 63
64 65 66 67 68 69 70
71 72 73 74 75 76 77
78 79 80 81 82 83 84

TODAY'S FOCUS

ACTION: Remember two phrases: "Stick to it and get through it," and "No, thank you." Use them whenever you need them!

WORKOUT

PHASE 3: STRENGTH 2

MENU PLAN

Take supplements: 1 to 2 grams omega-3s, multivitamin, and 1,000 IU vitamin D
Plus 1 serving of Greens+

Breakfast
Omelet Cup (page 181)
1 cup berries

Snack
1 hard-cooked egg
5 strawberries

Lunch
1 serving Quinoa Salad (page 229)

Snack
Post-Workout Shake (page 85)

Dinner
5 ounces cooked tilapia
Caprese Salad (page 102)

Day 69

TODAY'S FOCUS

ACTION: Are you recovering?
Your training programs have
stepped up a notch,
so make sure you are making
recovery and regeneration
a priority. If you have a hard
time increasing the weights or
pushing your intensity harder
than last time or doing more
with each workout, then you
may not have recovered fully
from the previous workout.
Do not ignore any kind of pain.
Usually when you first feel
a twinge, it is because a muscle
is too tight and pulling on the
joint. With some stretching and
foam rolling you can loosen
it up before it worsens. Listen
and give back to your body.

WORKOUT

PHASE 3: COMPLEX METABOLIC

MENU PLAN

*Take supplements: 1 to 2 grams omega-3s,
multivitamin, and 1,000 IU vitamin D*
Plus 1 serving of Greens+

. . . .

Breakfast
1 Ezekiel English muffin
1 tablespoon almond butter

Snack
2 pieces Laughing Cow light cheese
5 strawberries

Lunch
*1 Chicken Salad Wrap (page 171;
see Day 66)*

Snack
Post-Workout Shake (page 85)

Dinner
Tofu Stir-Fry (page 84)

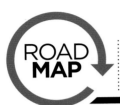

Day 70

PHASE 3

Week 10

57	58	59	60	61	62	63
64	65	66	67	68	69	70
71	72	73	74	75	76	77
78	79	80	81	82	83	84

TODAY'S FOCUS ✓

ACTION: Prepare in advance.
By now you know how important it is to plan ahead. It makes everything easier and sets you up for guaranteed success. With that in mind, let's plan ahead for the next week. Prepare your veggies and protein in advance, plan out times for your workouts, and be ready to tackle your week prepared.

WORKOUT 🏃

DAY OFF: Active Recovery
or complete day of rest.

MENU PLAN 🍴

Take supplements: 1 to 2 grams omega-3s, multivitamin, and 1,000 IU vitamin D
Plus 1 serving of Greens+

Breakfast
1 cup 2% Greek yogurt
½ cup fresh berries
2 tablespoons chopped raw almonds

Snack
A handful of raw almonds

Lunch
Asian Chicken Salad (page 94) and Sesame Dressing (page 95)

Snack
Post-Workout Shake (page 85)

Dinner
4 ounces cooked shrimp, 1 cup diced tomatoes, ¼ cup grated Parmesan cheese, and fresh basil

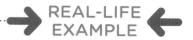
Wonder Woman

KRISTI MIRANDA > dropped from a size 18 to a size 6

I was in a really rough place. I was severely depressed, had all kinds of injuries, was on several medications, and I had just started raising my daughter completely on my own. I really believed I was weak, worthless, and incapable—I lost myself. My daughter inspires me and was the reason for my turning point.

It finally hit me that my daughter didn't know who I really was, who I used to be. Strong, smart, independent, and fun. After starting the Drop Two Sizes plan, I was feeling stronger and like I could actually handle all the challenges I was facing. The gym was a place where I felt supported, where I would work off stress and frustrations. I started to gradually feel better about myself and I realized I was a good person and a great mom.

I started to look for new challenges that would help me on my journey. One of my trainers at the gym suggested a powerlifting meet, so I decided to do it. Through my training I was lifting more and more weight, getting stronger and stronger—not only physically, but mentally and emotionally. At my first powerlifting competition, after I made my lift, my daughter came running up to me. She told me, "Mommy, you're just like Wonder Woman! When I grow up, can I be strong like you?" I almost burst into tears. She had no idea what that meant to me and on so many levels—she was watching me and I was sending all the right messages.

This journey has taught me I can accomplish ANYTHING I set my mind to. My biggest accomplishment by far is that I feel stronger than I ever have in my life. It has made me an even better parent and given me the power physically, mentally, and spiritually to handle anything life sends my way.

before   *after*

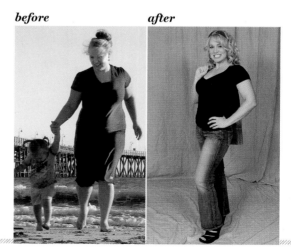

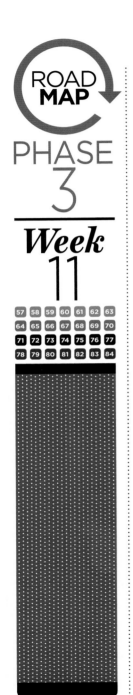

ROAD MAP

PHASE 3

Week 11

57	58	59	60	61	62	63
64	65	66	67	68	69	70
71	**72**	**73**	**74**	**75**	**76**	**77**
78	79	80	81	82	83	84

Welcome to Week Eleven!

As you head into this week, I want you to think ahead to another goal in the future that you can start to look forward to. As you know, this challenge doesn't end in 2 weeks! As focused as you should be on this plan, I want you to also let yourself dream and visualize what you want to accomplish beyond it. You're only 2 weeks away from your goal of dropping two sizes (or maybe more!).

Take time to think about the bigger picture. What will your next goal be? Will you run a 5-K? Or plan a beach vacation where you can rock a bikini for the first time in a while? Take a look at some of the inspiring stories in this book and think about how you will continue your new habits into the rest of your life.

Week Eleven Plan of Attack:

Let's return to the vow we discussed back in Chapter 3. Hopefully it has been a motivational tool for you throughout these past 10 weeks. Now, let's alter it so that it fits not only the rest of this plan, but the rest of your life:

"I vow that over the rest of my life, I will not step foot on a scale. I will not count calories. I will only use my clothing as measurement. I will fuel my body with the right foods and challenge myself with workouts. I promise that I will only say nice things to myself. I will trust that I know how to stay fit and healthy."

Week Eleven Grocery List

PRODUCE

- Berries
- Lemons
- Avocados (2)
- Beets
- Bell peppers
- Broccoli
- Cabbage
- Carrots, baby
- Celery
- Greens, mixed
- Onion, red
- Portobello mushroom (1)
- Spinach
- Tomatoes
- Cilantro (optional)
- Hummus

DAIRY & EGGS

- Cheese, feta (crumbled)
- Cheese, shredded
- Eggs
- Greek yogurt, 2% (plain)
- Milk, 2% (cow, soy, or almond)

BAKERY

- Corn tortillas
- Ezekiel tortilla

MEAT, DELI & SEAFOOD

- Chicken breasts, boneless, skinless (1 pound)
- Flank steak (about ⅓ pound)
- Mahi mahi or tilapia
- Salmon, wild-caught (6 ounces)
- Shrimp
- Turkey breast or buffalo, ground

GROCERY & PANTRY

- Ak-mak or RyKrisp crackers
- Almonds, raw
- Beans, black, canned (15 ounces)
- Broth, chicken or vegetable
- Oatmeal (rolled oats)
- Olives, black
- Salsa
- Whey protein powder

FROZEN

- Berries

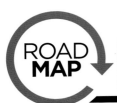

ROAD MAP

Day 71

PHASE
3

Week
11

57	58	59	60	61	62	63
64	65	66	67	68	69	70
71	**72**	**73**	**74**	**75**	**76**	**77**
78	79	80	81	82	83	84

TODAY'S FOCUS

Checkpoint: **Splurge Check**
Take inventory of your splurges. At this point you should have had no more than 30. What's your total? Flip back through your journal to figure out what your cravings are and how you've tackled them in the past.

WORKOUT

PHASE 3: STRENGTH 1

MENU PLAN

Take supplements: 1 to 2 grams omega-3s, multivitamin, and 1,000 IU vitamin D
Plus 1 serving of Greens+

Breakfast
1 cup cooked oatmeal (made with 2% milk)
1 cup fresh berries

Snack
1 hard-cooked egg
A handful of baby carrots

Lunch
Hummus and Veggie Wrap (page 172)

Snack
Post-Workout Shake (page 85)

Dinner
Turkey or buffalo burger on one grilled portobello mushroom topped with ½ avocado and spinach
Side Salad (page 83) and 1 tablespoon Homemade Vinaigrette (page 151)

Day 72

TODAY'S FOCUS ✓

Checkpoint: **Attitude Check**
With 2 weeks left, it's a good time to check your mind-set. Are you feeling good? Positive? Expecting to succeed? If you still have any doubts about your ability to reach your goals, review your journal and remember every moment you felt empowered and strong.

WORKOUT

DAY OFF: **Active Recovery,** optional 20-minute interval workout, or repeat this week's metabolic workout.

MENU PLAN

Take supplements: 1 to 2 grams omega-3s, multivitamin, and 1,000 IU vitamin D
Plus 1 serving of Greens+

. . . .

Breakfast
1 egg + 3 egg whites scrambled with 1 cup fresh vegetables and spinach

Snack
¼ cup raw almonds
1 bell pepper, sliced

Lunch
Chicken Pizza (page 150)
Side Salad (page 83) and 1 tablespoon Homemade Vinaigrette (page 151)

Snack
Post-Workout Shake (page 85)

Dinner
1 serving Black Bean Soup (page 97). Refrigerate the second serving for lunch on Day 76.)
Side Salad (page 83) and 1 tablespoon Homemade Vinaigrette (page 151)

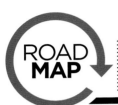
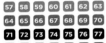

PHASE 3

Week 11

57	58	59	60	61	62	63
64	65	66	67	68	69	70
71	72	73	74	75	76	77
78	79	80	81	82	83	84

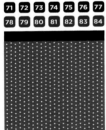

Day 73

TODAY'S FOCUS ✓

ACTION: Cut back on sodium.
Start to eliminate any foods with a lot of sodium, such as anything canned or packaged, processed deli meat (even if it's all natural), cottage cheese and other cheeses, and most nut butters (which have added salt). Cutting out some of these foods while drinking plenty of water will help you to drop any bloat in the final weeks of the plan.

WORKOUT

PHASE 3: STRENGTH 2

MENU PLAN

Take supplements: 1 to 2 grams omega-3s, multivitamin, and 1,000 IU vitamin D
Plus 1 serving of Greens+

Breakfast
1 cup cooked oatmeal (made with 2% milk)
1 cup fresh berries

Snack
1 hard-cooked egg
A handful of baby carrots

Lunch
Chicken and Avocado Salad (page 92)

Snack
Post-Workout Shake (page 85)

Dinner
6 ounces grilled shrimp
2 cups broccoli roasted with 2 teaspoons olive oil

Day 74

TODAY'S FOCUS

ACTION: Shed extra water weight.

Add in more asparagus, lemon in your water, cucumbers, and strawberries, and take extra vitamin C—these are all foods that naturally help you to drop any water you might be retaining, which will help the way your clothes fit and feel.

WORKOUT

DAY OFF: Active Recovery or complete day of rest.

MENU PLAN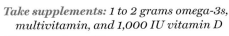

Take supplements: 1 to 2 grams omega-3s, multivitamin, and 1,000 IU vitamin D
Plus 1 serving of Greens+

. . . .

Breakfast
Smoothie: *1 cup 2% Greek yogurt, 1 cup berries*

Snack
½ cup hummus with celery sticks

Lunch
4 ounces grilled chicken
Beet Salad (page 112)

Snack
Post-Workout Shake (page 85)

Dinner
6 ounces wild-caught salmon (skin removed), grilled*

2 cups steamed or roasted vegetable of choice

*Sprinkle with chili powder or dry rub of choice and grill for 4 to 5 minutes per side.

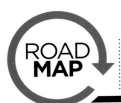

ROAD MAP

Day 75

PHASE **3**

Week 11

57	58	59	60	61	62	63
64	65	66	67	68	69	70
71	72	73	74	75	76	77
78	79	80	81	82	83	84

TODAY'S FOCUS ⊘

ACTION: Tune in to how great you feel.

You may have cut back on your splurges at this point, so you may have to say, "No, thank you" more than you are used to this weekend. For every uncomfortable moment you face, tune in to how great you are feeling overall. No amount of junk food or binge session will taste as good as you'll feel in your favorite clothes! Stay focused.

WORKOUT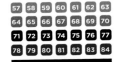

PHASE 3: STRENGTH 1

MENU PLAN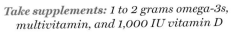

Take supplements: 1 to 2 grams omega-3s, multivitamin, and 1,000 IU vitamin D
Plus 1 serving of Greens+

Breakfast
1 cup cooked oatmeal (made with 2% milk)
1 cup fresh berries

Snack
¼ cup raw almonds
A handful of baby carrots

Lunch
Hummus and Veggie Wrap (page 98)

Snack
Post-Workout Shake (page 85)

Dinner
Steak Salad (see opposite)

Day 76

TODAY'S FOCUS

Checkpoint: **Sleep Check**
Are you getting enough shut-eye? Your training has stepped up this last phase, so it is even more important that you are getting enough sleep. Get into a ritual of hitting the sack at the same time each night and waking up at the same time each morning, aiming for at least 6 to 8 hours of sleep a night. Your body will thank you.

WORKOUT

PHASE 3: COUNTDOWN METABOLIC

MENU PLAN

Take supplements: 1 to 2 grams omega-3s, multivitamin, and 1,000 IU vitamin D
Plus 1 serving of Greens+

Breakfast
Smoothie: *1 cup 2% Greek yogurt, 1 cup berries*

Snack
*1 hard-cooked egg
A handful of baby carrots*

Lunch
*1 serving Black Bean Soup (page 97; see Day 72)
5 ak-mak or RyKrisp crackers
Side Salad (page 83) and 1 tablespoon Homemade Vinaigrette (page 151)*

Snack
Post-Workout Shake (page 85)

Dinner
*Beet Salad (page 112)
4 ounces cooked chicken or fish*

Steak Salad

5 ounces grilled flank steak (thinly sliced)

3 cups mixed greens

½ cup diced tomato

¼ cup crumbled feta cheese

1 tablespoon extra virgin olive oil

vinegar to taste

Combine all ingredients in a large bowl and dress with olive oil and vinegar.

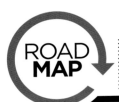

Day 77

Week
11

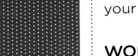

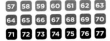

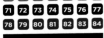

TODAY'S FOCUS ✓

ACTION: Building up your final week.

You're almost there! Stick to what you have been doing up until now. There is no reason to change anything drastically. A few final tips: Drink plenty of water, swap out your protein sources for fish this week as much as you can, avoid processed lunchmeats, watch your sodium, and look forward to your final moment of triumph!

WORKOUT

DAY OFF: Active Recovery or complete day of rest.

MENU PLAN 🍴

Take supplements: 1 to 2 grams omega-3s, multivitamin, and 1,000 IU vitamin D
Plus 1 serving of Greens+

Breakfast
1 cup cooked oatmeal (made with 2% milk)
1 cup fresh berries

Snack
¼ cup raw almonds
1 bell pepper, sliced

Lunch
Fish Tacos (page 218)

Snack
Post-Workout Shake (page 85)

Dinner
Chicken and Avocado Salad (page 92)

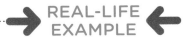
Her Morning Therapy

CYNDI MADIA > dropped three sizes in 12 weeks

After hearing about Drop Two Sizes, I knew this was a book for me—but what I didn't realize was that this little book was going to transform my life. Right away, I changed my eating habits, started drinking more water, and gave up my daily runs for a strength-training regimen. In just 8 weeks, I had to replace my old jeans with new ones because I had dropped two sizes! By the end of Week 12, I had dropped another.

I have met all my goals and continue to make new ones every month. I am a mom of two great kids who are active in school and sports, wife to a husband who works long hours, and I work full time. I don't have much free time; finding the time to work out is a challenge. I have made the commitment to get up extra early (5:30 a.m.) to do what I now consider my morning therapy.

I've gone down three jean sizes at this point (those new jeans I bought are now way too big!), my abs are tighter than ever, and my body is looking better than I thought it could at 40. And, best of all, I find it to be a fun experience!

before   *after*

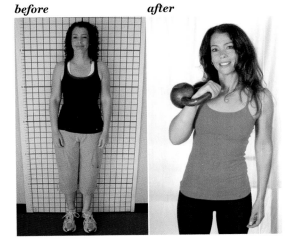

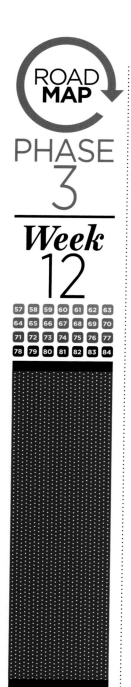

ROAD MAP

PHASE 3

Week 12

57	58	59	60	61	62	63
64	65	66	67	68	69	70
71	72	73	74	75	76	77
78	79	80	81	82	83	84

Week Twelve: The Final Countdown!

This is it! Let me just say that, quite frankly, you rock! You have worked so incredibly hard and committed to a powerful change that will benefit you in the short term and for the rest of your life. You've transformed your body and mind. Congratulations in advance—you're already a winner!

Some of you may have achieved your goal of dropping two sizes already, and I commend you for sticking to all 12 weeks of this challenge. As you know by now, it's not just following the plan that counts, but the repetition of positive habits that changes your outlook and transforms you for good. Start thinking about your next goal!

Week Twelve
Plan of Attack:

Celebrate! If you haven't already, plan something fun and special to do on the day you try on your clothes—a nice dinner out, dancing, a gathering of friends and family. It's a great way to keep focused this week and celebrate your success!

If you'd rather have a quiet celebration on your own, prepare a delicious, healthy dinner, and sit down and look back through your journal. Reflect on all that you have accomplished. Take note of all the times you struggled or faltered but ultimately persevered. You're amazing, inside and out! I'm so proud of you and I wish you a lifetime of looking and feeling absolutely fabulous.

Week Twelve Grocery List

PRODUCE

- Berries
- Lemons
- Limes
- Asparagus
- Bell peppers
- Broccoli
- Carrots, baby
- Cauliflower
- Celery
- Cucumber
- Eggplant
- Greens, mixed
- Spinach, baby
- Tomatoes
- Zucchini
- Herbs

DAIRY & EGGS

- Cheese, feta (crumbled)
- Cheese, shredded mozzarella
- Eggs
- Greek yogurt, 2% (plain)
- Milk, 2% (cow, soy, or almond)

BAKERY

- Ezekiel bread
- Ezekiel English muffins
- Ezekiel tortillas

MEAT, DELI & SEAFOOD

- Chicken breasts, boneless, skinless (2 pounds)
- Flank steak (about ¼ pound)
- Mahi mahi
- Orange roughy or halibut (optional)
- Pork tenderloin
- Salmon, wild-caught
- Tilapia
- Tuna, fresh

GROCERY & PANTRY

- Almonds, raw
- Barbecue sauce
- Beans, black (canned)
- Muir Glen Organic Marinara Sauce
- Oatmeal (rolled oats)
- Peanut butter, natural
- Quinoa
- Tuna, canned (water-packed)
- Whey protein powder

FROZEN

- Berries

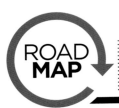
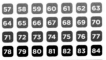

PHASE 3

Week 12

57	58	59	60	61	62	63
64	65	66	67	68	69	70
71	72	73	74	75	76	77
78	79	80	81	82	83	84

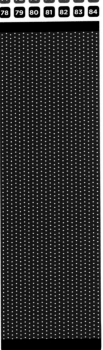

Day 78

TODAY'S FOCUS

ACTION: Finish stronger than you started.
Bring 100 percent of your energy and determination to every workout. Plan ahead for every day and finish this challenge stronger than you started it!

WORKOUT

PHASE 3: STRENGTH 2

MENU PLAN

Take supplements: 1 to 2 grams omega-3s, multivitamin, and 1,000 IU vitamin D
Plus 1 serving of Greens+

Breakfast
1 Ezekiel English muffin
2 tablespoons natural peanut butter

Snack
A handful of raw almonds
A handful of baby carrots

Lunch
3 ounces cooked chicken mixed with ¼ cup chopped celery, 1 tablespoon olive oil mayonnaise, and Dijon mustard to taste
3 cups mixed greens

Snack
Post-Workout Shake (page 85)

Dinner
5 ounces cooked chicken breast topped with ½ cup marinara sauce (Muir Glen Organic recommended) and thinly sliced bell pepper (to taste)
2 cups baby spinach topped with 2 teaspoons extra virgin olive oil and lemon juice to taste

Day 79

TODAY'S FOCUS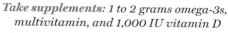

ACTION: Prime for your peak.
Commit to getting through this final week without a splurge. You can do it. This will prime you for your "peak" moment at your final Jeans Check. Remember to finish strong—you owe it to yourself.

WORKOUT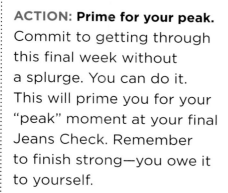

DAY OFF: Active Recovery, optional 20-minute interval workout, or repeat this week's metabolic workout.

MENU PLAN

Take supplements: 1 to 2 grams omega-3s, multivitamin, and 1,000 IU vitamin D
Plus 1 serving of Greens+

Breakfast
2-egg omelet with 1 cup vegetables and a handful of spinach
1 Ezekiel English muffin

Snack
A handful of raw almonds
1 bell pepper, sliced

Lunch
Chicken Salad Wrap (page 103)

Snack
Post-Workout Shake (page 85)

Dinner
4 ounces grilled flank steak
2 cups roasted or grilled vegetables (zucchini, eggplant, bell pepper)

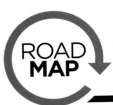

Day 80

PHASE 3

Week 12

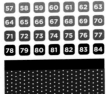

57	58	59	60	61	62	63
64	65	66	67	68	69	70
71	72	73	74	75	76	77
78	79	80	81	82	83	84

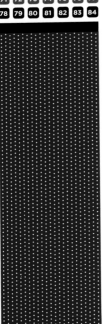

TODAY'S FOCUS

Checkpoint: Water Check

A week ago you eliminated most sodium from your diet and made sure you were drinking 64 ounces of water each day. Don't stop now!

WORKOUT

PHASE 3: STRENGTH 1

MENU PLAN

Take supplements: 1 to 2 grams omega-3s, multivitamin, and 1,000 IU vitamin D
Plus 1 serving of Greens+

Breakfast
1 cup cooked oatmeal (made with 2% milk)
2 tablespoons chopped raw almonds

Snack
1 hard-cooked egg
Sliced cucumber

Lunch
Quinoa Salad* (page 229)
3 ounces diced cooked chicken breast, canned (water-packed) tuna, or cooked fish

*Make a double batch for lunch on Day 84.

Snack
Post-Workout Shake (page 85)

Dinner
6 ounces cooked tilapia
1 cup chopped cauliflower, roasted with 2 teaspoons olive oil
Side Salad (page 83) and 1 tablespoon Homemade Vinaigrette (page 151)

Day 81

TODAY'S FOCUS

ACTION: Remember the little things.

Drinking one cup of green tea each day, taking your multi-vitamin, omega-3s, and vitamin D, and, of course, drinking water are the little things that will add up to a successful finish this week.

WORKOUT

DAY OFF: Active Recovery or complete day of rest.

MENU PLAN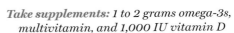

Take supplements: 1 to 2 grams omega-3s, multivitamin, and 1,000 IU vitamin D
Plus 1 serving of Greens+

Breakfast
1 cup 2% Greek yogurt
1 cup berries

Snack
3 ounces canned (water-packed) tuna with celery sticks

Lunch
Grilled Chicken Salad (page 104)

Snack
Post-Workout Shake (page 85)

Dinner
4 ounces grilled tuna
Side Salad (page 83) and 1 tablespoon Homemade Vinaigrette (page 151)

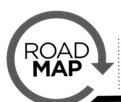

ROAD MAP

Day 82

PHASE
3

Week
12

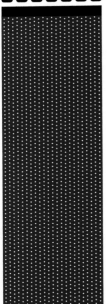

57	58	59	60	61	62	63
64	65	66	67	68	69	70
71	72	73	74	75	76	77
78	79	80	81	82	83	84

TODAY'S FOCUS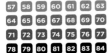

ACTION: Rev up your metabolism.
Today is your last strength workout of this program. Challenge yourself by using heavier weights on any of the exercises that are getting too easy. Really push your intensity to get your metabolism revved, and get ready to rock your jeans!

WORKOUT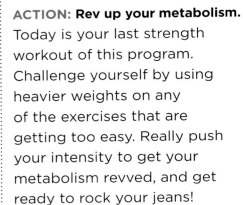

PHASE 3: STRENGTH 2

MENU PLAN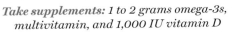

Take supplements: 1 to 2 grams omega-3s, multivitamin, and 1,000 IU vitamin D
Plus 1 serving of Greens+

Breakfast
2-egg omelet with 1 cup vegetables and spinach
½ Ezekiel English muffin

Snack
3 ounces cooked chicken
Sliced cucumbers

Lunch
1 slice Ezekiel bread with 2 tablespoons natural peanut butter
A handful of baby carrots

Snack
Post-Workout Shake (page 85)

Dinner
5 ounces grilled mahi mahi*
2 cups steamed chopped asparagus

*Brush with barbecue sauce and grill or roast.

Day 83

TODAY'S FOCUS

ACTION: Have a "me" day.
Have a "me" day (and don't feel guilty about it!). Buy a new top to go with your goal jeans or a new dress, see a movie, get a massage, or get your nails done. You deserve it as you head into the final days of the plan.

WORKOUT

PHASE 3: COMPLEX METABOLIC

MENU PLAN

Take supplements: 1 to 2 grams omega-3s, multivitamin, and 1,000 IU vitamin D
Plus 1 serving of Greens+

Breakfast
1 Ezekiel English muffin
1 egg, poached
1 cup berries

Snack
1 cup 2% Greek yogurt
Sliced cucumber

Lunch
3 ounces cooked chicken mixed with ½ cup chopped celery, 1 tablespoon olive oil mayonnaise, and Dijon mustard to taste
1 Ezekiel tortilla

Snack
Post-Workout Shake (page 85)

Dinner
5 ounces grilled salmon
2 cups baby spinach topped with 2 teaspoons extra virgin olive oil and lemon juice to taste

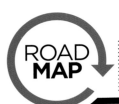
ROAD MAP

Day 84

PHASE 3

Week 12

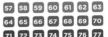
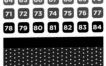

TODAY'S FOCUS ✓

***Checkpoint:* Final Jeans Check**

HERE WE GO. This is the day you have been working so hard for. I hope you planned a special date or activity so you can wear your outfit proudly and show off your stuff! You are amazing; you've accomplished a great deal over the past 12 weeks; and you're well on your way to a lifetime of feeling fabulous. Bravo!

WORKOUT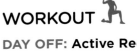

DAY OFF: Active Recovery or complete day of rest.

MENU PLAN 🍴

Take supplements: 1 to 2 grams omega-3s, multivitamin, and 1,000 IU vitamin D

Plus 1 serving of Greens+

Breakfast

2-egg omelet with 1 cup vegetables, such as broccoli

Snack

3 ounces cooked chicken
Celery sticks

Lunch

1 serving Quinoa Salad (page 229; see Day 80)

Snack

Post-Workout Shake (page 85)

Dinner

5 ounces grilled fish (orange roughy, halibut, or mahi mahi)

2 cups chopped asparagus, roasted with 2 teaspoons extra virgin olive oil

Baby Fat

CHERALYN GOECKERITZ > dropped two sizes in 12 weeks

Just when I was feeling good about the changes I had made and the shape I was in, along came a big surprise—baby number five! Over the course of my pregnancy, I kept up with my workouts as much as I could, but I gained 70 pounds and felt pretty discouraged.

But I accepted the challenge of getting my body back. Over the course of 8 weeks there will always be tough spots: sickness, travel, family issues, even injury.

I had them all this time. But life is never going to hand you 3 free months with no interruptions. The real challenge is to make it work in the middle of real life. And that's what I did. As life goes on the tough spots will keep popping up, but now I know I can handle them. After all, I didn't just want the jeans to fit for one fun picture day. I want these to be my new reality. So the healthy habits that got me here are my new reality as well.

With a brand new (beautiful!) baby, four other children, and a husband to look after, I still have to make my workouts and nutrition a priority. I make no excuses and try to be the best mom I can be. Nine months later I hit my lowest-ever weight and body fat percentage. I love my new jeans! I'm actually ready to go buy more! I got the best of both worlds—another wonderful child *and* a healthier, stronger body.

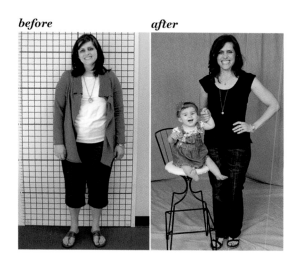

before   *after*

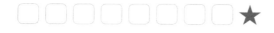

Congratu

You have completed the Drop Two Sizes challenge! Hopefully by now you're not only enjoying wearing clothes that are at least two sizes smaller than they were 12 weeks ago, but you're also enjoying the healthy habits you created over the past 84 days. This is an ongoing journey. You've learned how to maintain your new body—and your new clothing size—and you'll use these skills to keep them for life, even while enjoying an occasional splurge.

The idea behind this book is to eat and work out to live, not live to eat and work out. Your new habits should give you plenty of energy that you can channel into other goals and dreams you may have, which in turn will inspire you to remain fit and healthy so you can achieve them! One of my secrets to staying inspired is to help others—and all of you keep me going every day.

ations!

In addition to using the information in this book whenever you need a fitness or diet challenge, here are two important tips to keep you on track.

→ *Ditch your scale—really. At this point, your scale should be in the back of a closet or donated to Goodwill! The scale is not a measurement of your overall fitness or shape. Seriously, give your scale away! Don't get stuck in the old habit of stepping on the scale or watching those numbers. Use the clothes you chose for your Jeans Check instead—you may even have a whole new outfit now as your guide. Wear these clothes once a week to keep you accountable.*

→ *No more "fat" clothes. Remember the box of clothes you were supposed to toss at the beginning of this plan? If you haven't already, get rid of them! Those "fat pants" have no place in your closet. Scale your wardrobe down to one size—the size you now proudly wear.*

Life is too short not to look and feel your absolute best. I hope you have achieved that and more!

REFERENCES

Chapter 1

Campbell, W, M Crim, V Young, and W Evans. Increased energy requirements and changes in body composition with resistance training in older adults. *American Journal of Clinical Nutrition* 60 (1994): 167–75.

Carraça, EV, MN Silva, D Markland, PN Vieira, CS Minderico, LB Sardinha, and PJ Teixeira. Body image change and improved eating self-regulation in a weight management intervention in women. *Int J Behav Nutr Phys Act* 8:75 (July 18, 2011).

Lombard, C, A Deeks, D Jolly, HJ Teede, and Jean Hailes. Preventing weight gain: the baseline weight related behaviors and delivery of a randomized controlled intervention in community based women. *BMC Public Health* 2009 January 3; 9:2.

Pikosky, M, A Faigenbaum, W Westcott, and N Rodriguez. Effects of resistance training on protein utilization in healthy children. *Medicine and Science in Sports and Exercise* 34, no. 5 (2002): 820–27.

Pratley, R, B Nicklas, M Rubin, J Miller, A Smith, M Smith, B Hurley, and A Goldberg. Strength training increases resting metabolic rate and norepinephrine levels in healthy 50- to 65-year-old men. *Journal of Applied Physiology* 76 (1994): 133–37.

Ryttig, KR, H Flaten, and S Rössner. Long-term effects of a very low calorie diet (Nutrilett) in obesity treatment. A prospective, randomized, comparison between VLCD and a hypocaloric diet+behavior modification and their combination. *Int J Obesity Relat Met Disorder* 21, no. 7 (July 1997): 574–79.

Sumithran, Priya, LA Prendergast, E Delbridge, K Purcell, A Shulkes, Sc.D., A Kriketos, and J Proietto. Long-term persistence of hormonal adaptations to weight loss. *N Engl J Med* 2011; 365:1597–1604.

Teixeira, PJ, MN Silva, SR Coutinho, AL Palmeira, J Mata, PN Vieira, EV Carraça, TC Santos, and LB Sardinha. Mediators of weight loss and weight loss maintenance in middle aged women. *Obesity Journal* 18, no. 4 (April 2010): 725–35.

UNC Gillings School of Global Public Health, University of North Carolina at Chapel Hill with *SELF* magazine. Survey finds disordered eating behaviors among three out of four American Women. April 22, 2008.

Vesilind, Emili. "Fashion's Invisible Woman," *LA Times*, March 1, 2009.

Westcott, Wayne. Increased muscle = increased resting metabolic rates = increased weight loss, 2011.

Chapter 2

Brodie, DA, and PD Slade (1988). The relationship between body-image and body-fat in adult women. *Psychological Medicine* 18 (1988): 623–31. doi:10.1017/S0033291700008308

Cruz P, BD Johnson, SC Karpinski, KA Limoges, BA Warren, KD Olsen, VK Somers, MD Jensen, MM Clark, and F Lopez-Jimenez . Validity of weight loss to estimate improvement in body composition in individuals attending a wellness center. *Obesity* (Silver Spring) 19, no. 11 (November 2011): 2274–79. doi: 10.1038/oby.2011.102. Epub 2011 May 12.

Donnelly, et al. Muscle hypertrophy with large-scale weight loss and resistance training. *Am J Clin Nutr.* 58, no. 4 (October 1993): 561–65.

Fox, Kate. Mirror, mirror: a summary of research findings on body image. Social Issues Research Centre, 1997.

Han, TS, E Gates, E Truscott, and MEJ Lean. Clothing size as an indicator of adiposity, ischaemic heart disease and cardiovascular risks. *Journal of Human Nutrition and Dietetics* 18 (2005): 423–30. doi: 10.1111/j.1365-277X.2005.00646.x

Hughes, LA, LJ Schouten, RA Goldbohm, PA van den Brandt, and MP Weijenberg. Self-reported clothing size as a proxy measure for body size. *Epidemiology* 20, no. 5 (September 2009): 673–76.

Ross, R, I Janssen, J Dawson, AM Kungl, JL Kuk, SL Wong, TB Nguyen-Duy, S Lee, K Kilpatrick, and R Hudson. Exercise-induced reduction in obesity and insulin resistance in women: a randomized controlled trial. *Obes Res.* 12, no. 5 (May 2004):789–98.

Ryttig, KR, H Flaten, and S Rössner. Long-term effects of a very low calorie diet (Nutrilett) in obesity treatment. A prospective, randomized, comparison between VLCD and a hypocaloric diet+behavior modification and their combination. *Int J Obesity Relat Met Disorder* 21, no. 7 (July 1997): 574–79.

Stiegler, P, and A Cunliffe. The role of diet and exercise for the maintenance of fat-free mass and resting metabolic rate during weight loss. *Sports Med.* 36, no. 3 (2006): 239–62.

Chapter 5

Conlon, KE, J Ehrlinger, RP Eibach, AW Crescioni, JL Alquist, MA Gerend, and GR Dutton. Eyes on the prize: the longitudinal benefits of goal focus on progress toward a weight loss goal. *J Exp Soc Psychol*. 47, no. 4 (July 2011):853–55.

Gilliat-Wimberly, M, MM Manore, K Woolf, PD Swan, and SS Carroll. Effects of habitual physical activity on the resting metabolic rates and body compositions of women aged 35 to 50 years. *J Am Diet Assoc*. 101, no. 10 (October 2001): 1181–88.

Chapter 7

Acheson, KJ, A Blondel-Lubrano, S Oguey-Araymon, M Beaumont, S Emady-Azar, C Ammon-Zufferey, I Monnard, S Pinaud, C Nielsen-Moennoz, and L Bovetto. Protein choices targeting thermogenesis and metabolism. *Am J Clin Nutr*. 93, no. 3 (March 2011): 525–34; Epub January 12, 2011.

Bopp, MJ, DK Houston, L Lenchik, L Easter, SB Kritchevsky, and BJ Nicklas. Lean mass loss is associated with low protein intake during dietary-induced weight loss in postmenopausal women. *J Am Diet Assoc*. 108, no. 7 (July 2008):1216–20.

Boutcher, SH. High-intensity intermittent exercise and fat loss. *J Obe*. 2011:868305. Epub November 24, 2010.

Caron-Jobin, M, AS Morisset, A Tremblay, C Huot, D Légaré, and A Tchernof. Elevated serum 25(OH)D concentrations, vitamin D, and calcium intakes are associated with reduced adipocyte size in women. *Obesity* (Silver Spring) 19, no. 7 (July 2011):1335–41. doi: 10.1038/oby.2011.90. Epub April 28, 2011.

Harvie, MN, M Pegington, MP. Mattson, J Frystyk, B Dillon, G Evans, J Cuzick, SA Jebb, B Martin, RG Cutler, TG Son, S Maudsley, OD Carlson, JM Egan, A Flyvbjerg, and A Howell. The effects of intermittent or continuous energy restriction on weight loss and metabolic disease risk markers: a randomised trial in young overweight women. *Int J Obes* (Lond). 35, no. 5 (May 2011): 714–27.

Josse, AR, SA Atkinson, MA Tarnopolsky, and SM Phillips. Increased consumption of dairy foods and protein during diet- and exercise-induced weight loss promotes fat mass loss and lean mass gain in overweight and obese premenopausal women. *J Nutr*. 141, no. 9 (September 2011): 1626–34. Epub July 20, 2011.

Paoli, A, F Pacelli, AM Bargossi, G Marcolin, S Guzzinati, M Neri, A Bianco, and A Palma. Effects of three distinct protocols of fitness training on body composition, strength and blood lactate. *J Sports Med Phys Fitness* 50, no. 1 (March 2010): 43–51.

Riggs, AJ, BD White, and SS Gropper. Changes in energy expenditure associated with ingestion of high protein, high fat versus high protein, low fat meals among underweight, normal weight, and overweight females. *Nutr J*. 6 (November 12, 2007): 40.

Rodacki, CL, AL Rodacki, G Pereira, K Naliwaiko, I Coelho, D Pequito, and LC Fernandes. Fish-oil supplementation enhances the effects of strength training in elderly women. *Am J Clin Nutr*. 95, no. 2 (February 2012): 428–36. Epub January 4, 2012.

Shaw, K, P O'Rourke, C Del Mar, and J Kenardy. Psychological interventions for overweight or obesity. *Cochrane Database System Rev*. 2 (April 18, 2005): CD003818.

Shellock, FG, and WE, Prentice. Warming-up and stretching for improved physical performance and prevention of sports-related injuries. *Sports Med*. 2, no. 4 (July–August 1985): 267–78.

Shingo, Takada, Koichi Okita, Tadashi Suga, Masashi Omokawa, Tomoyasu Kadoguchi, Noriteru, Morita, Masahiro Horiuchi, Masashige Takahashi, Takashi Yokota, Kagami Hirabayashi, Shintaro Kinugawa, and Hiroyuki Tsutsui. High-metabolic stress during resistance exercise might provide muscle hypertrophy and strength increase even with low-mechanical stimulus. American College of Sports Medicine, June 2010.

Smith, GI, P Atherton, DN Reeds, BS Mohammed, D Rankin, MJ Rennie, and B Mittendorfer. Dietary omega-3 fatty acid supplementation increases the rate of muscle protein synthesis in older adults: a randomized controlled trial. *Am J Clin Nutr*. 93, no. 2 (February 2011): 402–12. Epub December 15, 2010.

Smith, GI, P Atherton, DN Reeds, BS Mohammed, D Rankin, MJ Rennie, and B Mittendorfer. Omega-3 polyunsaturated fatty acids augment the muscle protein anabolic response to hyperinsulinaemia-hyperaminoacidaemia in healthy young and middle-aged men and women. *Clin Sci* (Lond). 121, no. 6 (September 2011): 267–78.

Trapp, EG, DJ Chisholm, J Freund, and SH Boutcher. The effects of high-intensity intermittent exercise training on fat loss and fasting insulin levels of young women. *Int J Obes* (Lond) 32, no. 4 (April 2008):684–91. Epub January 15, 2008.

Wyatt, HR, GK Grunwald, CL Mosca, ML Klem, RR Wing, and JO Hill. Long-term weight loss and breakfast in subjects in the National Weight Control Registry. *Obesity Research* 10 (2002): 78–82; doi: 10.1038/oby.2002.13.

INDEX

Boldface page references indicate photographs. <u>Underscored</u> references indicate boxed text.

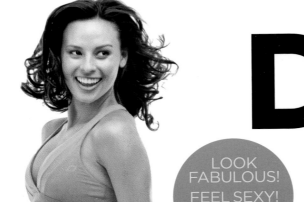

DROP TWO SIZES

LOOK FABULOUS! FEEL SEXY! LOVE YOUR BODY!

THE DVD PROGRAM

Get the workout of your life with America's #1 trainer, RACHEL COSGROVE! When you follow along to the *Drop Two Sizes DVD Program,* Rachel motivates you to give your all, from start to finish— for a fitter, sexier, more confident YOU.

YOU can work out with RACHEL COSGROVE!

The complete 12-week DROP TWO SIZE program is now on DVD!

→ *In the 6-DVD program, Rachel will coach you through every single exercise, the same way she would if you hire her as your personal trainer.*

→ *PLUS! the Drop Two Sizes DVD Program is specially designed so you can do every routine with just dumbbel a sturdy step, and a foam roll.*

→ *It's like having America's #1 trainer in your living room!*

→ *Schedule your appointment with Rachel today to shrink your hips, flatten your belly, and tone every inch of your bo*

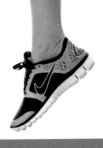

RODAL